General Preface to the Series

Because it is no longer possible for one textbook to cover the whole field of biology while remaining sufficiently up to date, the Institute of Biology has sponsored this series so that teachers and students can learn about significant developments. The enthusiastic acceptance of 'Studies in Biology' shows that the books are providing authoritative views of biological topics.

The features of the series include the attention given to methods, the selected list of books for further reading and, wherever possible, suggestions for practical work.

Readers' comments will be welcomed by the Education Officer of the Institute.

1980

Institute of Biology
41 Queen's Gate
London SW7 5HU

Preface

The immune system, as developed during the course of vertebrate evolution, is of crucial importance to the health of mankind. Its fascination, however, spreads far beyond the confines of medical science. In its capacity to distinguish between self and non-self it provides for the biologist a unique example of cellular recognition, reflecting a capacity which may be universal among living organisms and which has become adapted to serve many different functions. Vertebrate immunity also provides the cell biologist with insights into the regulation of cellular physiology and cellular interactions while the production of antibody serves as a model for protein synthesis in general. Elsewhere in biology, antibodies themselves have proved a useful if not essential tool in taxonomy, histochemistry and in radio-immunoassays for blood concentrations of hormones and other molecules.

The purpose of this book is to provide a brief survey of vertebrate immune mechanisms, setting them in their wider biological context. Because immunological research is moving very rapidly, new questions are raised with every old question that is answered and, rather than indulge in too much speculation, some arguments are left open-ended in the text. Inevitably, also, some aspects of immunology will be left out, particularly since the bias is biological rather than clinical. Nevertheless it is hoped that this introduction will be useful not only to biologists but also to medical students who wish to understand the fundamentals of the subject.

I should like to record my thanks to my colleague, Dr H. S. Micklem, for his help in the preparation of this book.

Edinburgh, 1980

C.J.I.

Contents

£3.75

The Institute of Biology's
Studies in Biology no. 128

Immunobiology

Christopher J. Inchley

Lecturer in Zoology,
University of Edinburgh

Edward Arnold

First published 1981
by Edward Arnold (Publishers) Limited
41 Bedford Square, London WC1 3DQ

British Library Cataloguing in Publication Data

Inchley, Christopher J
Immunobiology. – (Institute of Biology. Studies in biology; ISSN 0537–9024).
1. Immunology 2. Vertebrates – Physiology
I. Title II. Series
596′.02′95 QR181

ISBN 0–7131–2808–9

Printed and bound in Great Britain at
The Camelot Press Ltd, Southampton

1 Immunological Strategy

1.1 Phagocytic cells and immunity

All multicellular animals are equipped with defensive mechanisms which afford protection against invasion of the body by micro-organisms or other parasites. In the simplest Metazoa, these defences may depend almost entirely on phagocytic cells, whose major function is to engulf and digest foreign organisms or their harmful secretions. On the other hand, in higher animals, complex immune systems are found which involve a variety of cell types together with specialized organs such as the vertebrate spleen, bone marrow, thymus and liver. Despite the evolution of these additional mechanisms, however, phagocytes remain a fundamental means of defence throughout the Metazoa as well as providing an immunological link between the most lowly and the most advanced groups. While their role in immunity has become augmented during the course of evolution, mammalian phagocytes still share with those of the sponges and the coelenterates the basic properties of ingestion and digestion of foreign or unwanted cells, particles or molecules.

Phagocytic cells provide what has come to be known as *natural* or *non-specific* immunity. In the first demonstration of immunity in action at the cellular level, this particular system was discovered by the Russian biologist Metchnikoff in the 1880s, when he noticed that small splinters, implanted into molluscs and other invertebrates, were surrounded and engulfed by wandering amoeboid cells. Among the mammals, non-specific immunity is provided by two families of phagocytic cells which are related in that they both derive, in adults, from stem cells in the bone marrow. The first of these groups is comprised of motile, blood-borne *monocytes* (Fig. 1–1) and relatively sessile *macrophages* which are found in organs such as the lungs, spleen and liver. The second category also consists of blood-borne cells known as *granulocytes,* or sometimes as polymorphonuclear leukocytes (often shortened to polymorphs), the former name owing its origin to the prominent cytoplasmic inclusions which are characteristic of this class (Fig. 1–1). On the basis of their staining characteristics, granulocytes are further divided into neutrophils (the most frequent), eosinophils and basophils. The roles of these two families of phagocyte in immunity are often interlinked. For instance, if a localized infection becomes established in the skin, granulocytes quickly find their way to the spot and engulf large numbers

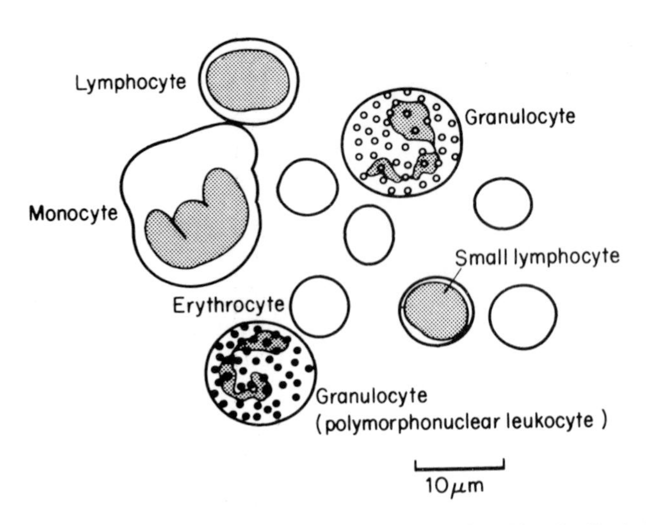

Fig. 1–1 Diagram to show the types of leukocyte (white blood cells) involved in immune mechanisms in mammals. Some red cells are given for comparison. Normally they are far more numerous, about 5×10^6 mm^{-3} compared with 5×10^3 mm^{-3} for leukocytes.

of bacteria, often succumbing in the process and forming pus. At a later stage, monocytes enter the lesion and engulf and digest both surviving bacteria and the remains of other cells, a sort of mopping-up operation which limits tissue damage and brings the infection to a halt.

The term 'non-specific immunity' in this context derives from the fact that phagocytic cells show no inherent specificity for foreign material. Any phagocyte is potentially able to recognize and respond to any foreign cell or particle. This characteristic stands in contrast to the high degree of specificity which is associated with those cells, the *lymphocytes,* which mediate the other major category of immunity, *acquired immunity.*

1.2 Lymphocytes

Lymphocytes are small to medium-sized cells, often with very small quantities of cytoplasm (Fig. 1–1), which are found in the blood stream and the lymphoid tissues of the body (see Chapter 4 for a detailed discussion of their characteristics and behaviour). Like phagocytes they are derived in mammals from stem cells in the bone marrow. The cellular basis of acquired immunity has been exhaustively investigated among the vertebrates, since it is characteristic of this group of animals. However, immune mechanisms which show certain similarities to vertebrate acquired immunity have been discovered in some invertebrate phyla, and it remains of great interest to determine whether lymphocytes have an evolutionary history which extends back into the protochordates and beyond; and, indeed, whether any analogue of lymphocytes exists in protostomate invertebrates such as the annelids or arthropods.

The functional feature which best distinguishes lymphocytes from phagocytes is the fact that each lymphocyte normally responds to one foreign agent, or *antigen*, only. Hence the alternative term, *specific immunity*. The complete spectrum of specific immune responses in vertebrates is due to the provision of a large population of lymphocytes, only a small proportion of which will react to any one antigen. It is also a property of lymphocytes that having once encountered an antigen, they or their descendants are capable of a more rapid and more efficient *secondary response* if they encounter it a second time. The system of specific immunity thus exhibits immunological memory.

The characteristics of immunological memory have been recognized since the time of the Greeks, when it was appreciated that individuals who recovered from smallpox were unlikely to suffer again from the disease. Crude immunization procedures against smallpox were current in the seventeenth century, and in the late eighteenth century Jenner showed that immunization with the agent causing benign cowpox (the virus *Vaccinia*) protected against the more virulent, but antigenically related, smallpox (*Variola*). The property of immunological memory is the basis of all immunization procedures against bacterial and viral infections in man and domestic animals.

1.3 Antibodies and graft rejection: two sorts of immunity

Acquired immunity in vertebrates takes two distinct forms (Fig. 1–2), and it is now known that these are mediated by separate families of cell, commonly known as B- and T-lymphocytes (see Chapters 4 and 5). The first of these systems is *humoral immunity* in which B-lymphocytes, stimulated by contact with an antigen, produce daughter cells which secrete proteins with the capacity to bind specifically to that antigen. These proteins are called *antibodies*. Their production can be initiated by viruses, bacteria, or bacterial secretions such as tetanus or diphtheria toxins. The earliest clear demonstration of the presence of blood-borne (humoral) factors capable of protecting against disease was in 1891 when von Behring injected a young diphtheria patient with serum from

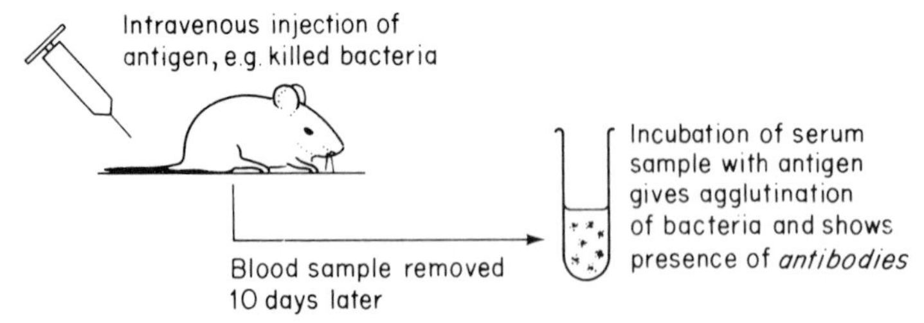

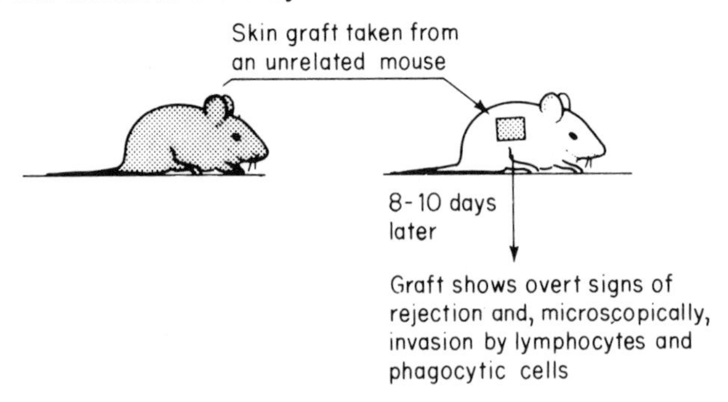

Fig. 1–2 Two sorts of acquired immunity. Humoral immunity involves production of antibodies by lymphocytes and is the typical response to systemic infections or inoculation with bacteria, viruses of foreign proteins. Cell-mediated immunity involves the direct destruction of foreign grafts, but the same mechanism may be activated following infection by intracellular parasites, or in some allergies.

an immunized sheep. The child recovered, and von Behring was awarded the first Nobel Prize for Medicine.

On the other hand, certain immune responses can occur which, although specific, do not involve antibodies. This is true, for instance, of the rejection of transplants of some foreign tissues such as skin; here, lymphocytes can kill cells of the graft by direct contact. Although antibodies *may* be produced at the same time, they are not necessary for graft rejection. As a consequence, this form of response is known as *cell-mediated immunity*. As well as graft rejection it also embraces certain hypersensitivity reactions (allergies), and the response to some intracellular parasites such as the tubercle bacillus.

Both humoral and cell-mediated types of immunity exhibit the specificity and generation of memory which are characteristic of acquired immunity. Thus a secondary antibody response is usually characterized by more rapid synthesis of antibody and, frequently, higher antibody concentrations in the blood, while a second skin graft is rejected more rapidly than a previous one from the same donor.

1.4 Relationship of natural and acquired immunity

Although natural and acquired forms of immunity rely primarily on different cell populations in the vertebrates, a close working relationship has become established between them. For instance, a major biological function of anti-bacterial antibodies is to improve the rate of phagocytosis of bacteria, particularly those such as species of *Pneumococcus* whose polysaccharide coat renders them resistant to ingestion by phagocytes. This function has been aided by the evolution of receptor sites within the macrophage plasma membrane. These can either bind antibodies directly or an ancillary molecule, one of a series of serum proteins which are activated following antigen – antibody binding. A summary of these interactions, and their role in phagocytosis is given in the next chapter, in Fig. 2–2. Other interactions between phagocytes and lymphocytes will be dealt with at a later stage.

The two cell populations, phagocyte and lymphocyte, also have a common feature in that they are able to distinguish what is antigenic or foreign: to tell 'self' from 'non-self'. A sensitive recognition system is absolutely fundamental to both types of immunity. Although, as will be seen, the molecular mechanisms for recognition differ between the two cell types, they probably both represent adaptations of a feature which is essential for successful multicellular life – a system of cell surface molecules which allows recognition and interaction between cells and hence the proper organization of the body into tissues and organs.

2 Evolution of Recognition Mechanisms

2.1 Cell interactions and recognition mechanisms

Recognition of foreign-ness is a cellular characteristic of most living organisms, and is certainly not confined to the immune systems of higher animals. The process of fertilization, for instance, well illustrates the need for cellular recognition mechanisms, and these may be found to operate before gamete fusion in both plants and animals. Among the angiosperms molecular mechanisms have been discovered which prevent both interspecific fertilization and, in some families, self-fertilization; in both instances pollen tube development is inhibited or restricted as a consequence of some recognition event (see HESLOP-HARRISON, 1978). Similar mechanisms operate during mating fusions in Protozoa such as *Paramecium*, and are equally important in metazoan species such as *Hydra* or *Nereis* where gametes are simply shed into the aquatic surroundings, and must be able to 'distinguish' those of the same species from the great variety of gametes which they may encounter. Even in higher animals where internal fertilization and behavioural isolating mechanisms serve to prevent interspecific gamete contact, the molecular mechanisms of gamete recognition still persist.

In a similar way, cellular recognition mechanisms are of great importance in all multicellular animals in determining the orderly development and arrangement of tissues and organs. This is particularly true during embryogenesis, where a great deal of cell movement and redistribution occurs, but it also applies during adult life, and lymphocytes themselves are a good example of cells whose re-circulation and tissue distribution are both carefully regulated (see section 4.5). The proper organization of the body, which can easily be taken for granted, would be most unlikely without the specific interactions which determine cell behaviour.

Interactions of this sort, at the level of cell–cell contact, have been best worked out in embryonic systems, and one of the more interesting results shows a parallel between the behaviour of dissociated tissues from vertebrate embryos (usually the chick) and the behaviour of dissociated sponge cells. Sponges are a sort of half-way house between colonial and true multicellular organization, and represent an evolutionary byway, but if their tissues are dissociated they show the ability to reform by reaggregation of the isolated cells. It has long been established that the reaggregation is species specific, and that if cell suspensions from two separate species are mixed, then the cells sort themselves out according to their original colonies. Within each colony there is also some sorting out according to cell type. Likewise, with the chick, if two embryonic tissues (such as liver and neural retina) are dissociated and their cells then mixed, reaggregation takes place, but also sorting out, so that the reforming complexes are specific for one or another of the tissues involved (Fig. 2–1).

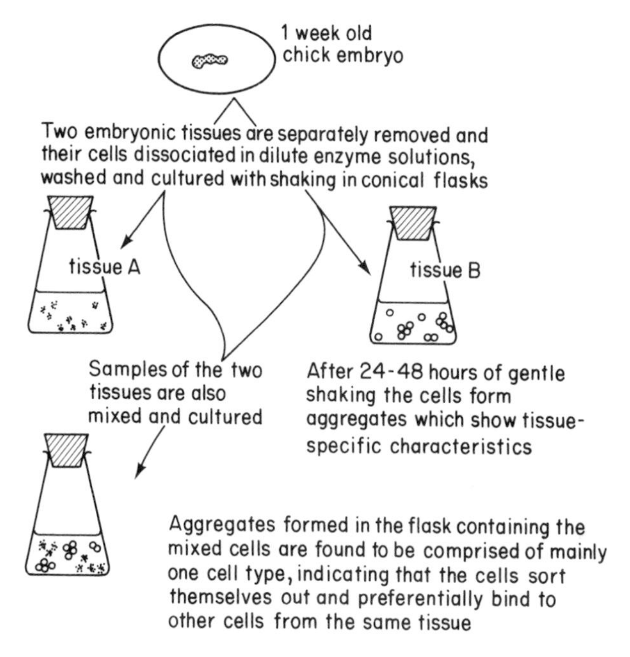

Fig. 2–1 Reaggregation and sorting out of mixed-tissue suspensions from chick embryos. Tissues used in these studies have included liver, retina, kidney, skin and limb-bud.

Reaggregation in both sponge and chick embryo systems is promoted by soluble factors which bind to tissue-specific receptor sites on the cell surfaces. There is not complete agreement at present as to the molecular nature of the factors involved, but it is clear that they have the common property of allowing 'like' cells to bind together while excluding 'unlike' cells. Although certain tissues are particularly amenable to this sort of experiment, it is not unreasonable to suggest that the integrity of many different tissues is due to this type of mechanism.

Whatever the details of the mechanisms involved, it is apparent that, from the earliest multicellular animals, cells have possessed surface molecules with the capacity to bind to ligands (either molecules or other cells), and to respond to this interaction in a specific way. With the evolution of more complex systems these mechanisms have multiplied to form, for instance, the basis of many endocrine systems (those involving polypeptide hormones), neurochemical transmission at synapses or neuro-muscular junctions, host-parasite specificities and so on. It is against this sort of background that the evolution of immune systems must be seen, and it should be said that a number of theoretical attempts have been made to explain the origins of immune recognition, particularly with respect to lymphocytes, in terms of pre-existing cell surface molecules with a tissue-recognition function. From these, receptors for foreign antigens might have evolved.

2.2 Evolutionary origins of vertebrate immunity

Mechanisms of acquired immunity can be traced back through the vertebrate line to the most primitive group, the jawless fish of the class Agnatha, represented in modern times only by the hagfish and the lamprey. In these animals we apparently see the beginnings of a system which increases in complexity throughout vertebrate evolution (see, for instance, section 4.4) and which gives rise to the mammalian system described in outline in the last chapter.

Lymphocytes are found in both hagfish and lamprey, but it is only in the latter species that these cells are organized into 'tissues' in the form of gut associated aggregates, particularly in the gill pouches, which may be the precursors of thymus and spleen. Both species are capable of rejecting tissue grafts and both are now known to be capable of making specific antibody molecules which appear to be related to one particular class of antibody found in jawed vertebrates and known as IgM (see Chapter 3). However antibody production in the hagfish in particular is not the physiologically straightforward affair that it is in mammals since the animal must be maintained at the near-lethal temperature of 18°C and repeatedly immunized before antibody molecules appear. It is difficult to see the adaptive advantage of a defence system which only comes into play at quite unnatural temperatures, quite apart from the means by which it could have been selected in the evolutionary sense. As a consequence some workers have suggested that the mechanisms of graft rejection preceded that by which antibodies are manufactured and secreted.

Although graft rejection is a feature of some invertebrate groups, the

Agnatha represent a true turning point in the evolution of immune mechanisms. While, in their possession of lymphocytes and antibodies, they foreshadow the more complex systems of higher vertebrates, they also show a variety of non-specific mechanisms which are more characteristic of the non-chordate phyla and to which we should briefly turn our attention.

2.3 Mechanisms of invertebrate immunity

As was indicated in Chapter 1, the characteristic immune effector cell in invertebrate phyla is the phagocyte, often referred to in this context as a haemocyte or an amoebocyte. This cell shows two characteristic responses to foreign material, phagocytosis and encapsulation, and together these provide an efficient defence against micro-organisms or their secretions and against invasion by metazoan parasites.

Phagocytosis proceeds in a similar manner to that shown by vertebrate phagocytes, and depends first on adhesion, for example of a bacterium to the cell membrane. While phagocytic cells can bind micro-organisms directly, particularly by interactions between carbohydrate chains on the two cell membranes, soluble factors known as *opsonins* are found in both vertebrates and higher invertebrates, and characteristically these promote adhesion and subsequent ingestion.

Among the vertebrates, some classes of antibody molecule and one of the components of the complement system (see section 3.5) are especially effective as opsonins, partly because some phagocytes have evolved specific cell membrane receptors for these molecules (Fig. 2–2). Factors which serve the same function have been identified in the body fluids of molluscs and arthropods in particular, but chemically these molecules seem to bear little relationship to their vertebrate counterparts. They are usually non-inducible substances, found in the body fluids of normal (un-immunized) animals, protein in nature but of variable size. Although they are clearly not antibodies, they frequently show the experimental property of being able to agglutinate bacteria or vertebrate red blood cells, sometimes with a high degree of specificity. The adhesiveness by which these natural agglutinins bind to recognized sites on the surface of, say, bacteria is undoubtedly of functional importance; for example, the mollusc *Aplysia* (the sea hare) is able to clear from its body fluids by phagocytosis those species of bacteria for which it possesses natural agglutinins, while bacteria for which no agglutinins exist can survive in the circulation.

It is clear that in some situations opsonins such as these are important for effective phagocytosis. However, experiments in which phagocytes are cultured in artificial media have shown that, for many organisms, opsonins added to the culture enhance phagocytic activity, but are not

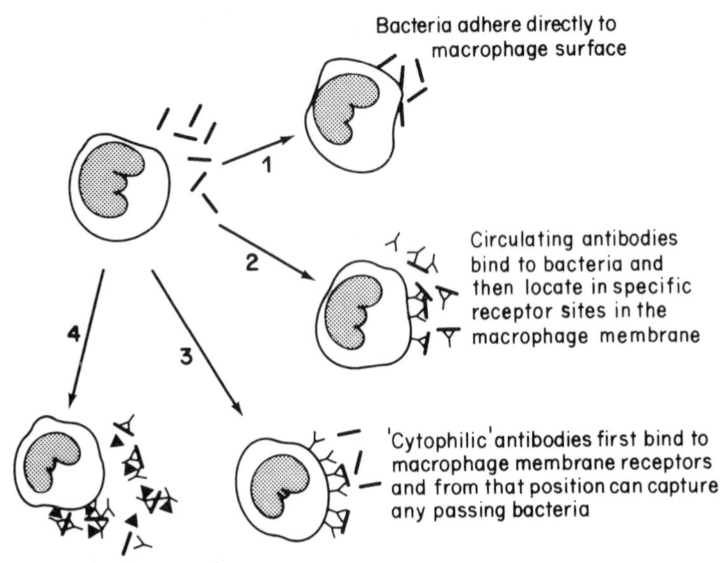

Fig. 2–2 Phagocytosis and opsonins in vertebrates. Macrophage membranes contain a number of receptor sites for molecules whose attachment to antigen thus improves phagocytosis. Not all antibodies are cytophilic or can fix complement, but a straightforward coat of antibody can often neutralize strong electrostatic charges on bacterial surfaces and make them more easily ingested.

essential for it. These observations agree with the evolutionary appearance of phagocytic cells in groups such as the sponges, before the development of vascular systems and of body fluids.

A further interesting feature of phagocytic activity in many invertebrate groups is the expulsion from the body of cells carrying ingested material. Thus in sponges, erythrocyte–laden amoebocytes have been observed to migrate to the excurrent canals, while in molluscs, micro-organisms may be removed by migration of phagocytes across epithelia to the exterior, as well as by normal intracellular digestion.

The second characteristic defence activity of invertebrate phagocytes is encapsulation, a response which may follow invasion by parasites, but which may also be experimentally induced by transplantation, for example, of nervous tissue or even small lengths of nylon into the haemocoel of insects. Encapsulation starts as a clustering of haemocytes around the foreign organism or tissue, but the cells eventually die, the tissue mass becoming first fibrous and then calcified. Isolation of the enclosed material thus becomes complete.

It is evident then that the invertebrate phyla have a well developed and versatile defense system based on phagocytic cells, but which may receive support from blood-borne opsonins in the higher groups. As in vertebrates, phagocytes are also responsible for the ingestion and removal of old or unwanted 'self' tissues. This is seen, for instance, in the insects during metamorphosis, but it is also a feature of lower groups and is found even in freshwater sponges where the flagellated cells of the free-swimming larva are phagocytosed when it adopts a sessile way of life. With the exception of encapsulation the general properties of phagocytic cells extend throughout the animal kingdom and, by and large, the system in invertebrates is as capable of discriminating between self and unwanted material as are the phagocytes of vertebrates.

2.4 Acquired responses in invertebrates

In addition to the mechanisms described above, a number of inducible or acquired responses have been identified among the invertebrates and some of these show features which are typically associated with lymphocyte-mediated mechanisms in vertebrates, for example, some sort of memory. The evolutionary relationship between these invertebrate forms of immunity and specific immunity in vertebrates is a biological question of considerable interest. However it must be remembered that the animal family tree split at a very early stage into two major lines, the deuterostomes, of which the echinoderms and the chordates are the best known phyla, and the protostomes which contain the molluscs, annelids and arthropods among other groups. There is only the most distant relationship then between higher invertebrates, as represented by insects, crustacea and arachnids, and the various vertebrate groups. Any similarities in their immune systems must either be due to the retention in both lines of primitive but worthwhile features, as seems to be the case with phagocytic cells, or to the evolution on more than one occasion of mechanisms which serve the same function. Taking the animal kingdom as a whole, this has certainly been the case with flight, air-breathing, and with the development of the segmented body plan which we see in chordates on the one hand and annelids and arthropods on the other. It may equally be true of the graft-rejection mechanisms which these same groups display.

Although molecules similar to vertebrate antibodies have not been isolated from the body fluids of invertebrates, a number of humoral factors have been discovered which have a role in immunity, including the natural agglutinins mentioned above. While the agglutinins are generally not inducible, others of these substances are. However close investigation shows a number of important differences between their induction and antibody synthesis.

One of the best studied molecules in this respect is a factor which was first identified after infection of the insect *Oncopiltus fasciatus* (the milk weed bug) with cultures of the bacterium *Pseudomonas aeruginosa*. It was found that a bacteriolytic agent was rapidly released into the haemolymph, its appearance after only four hours standing in marked contrast to the relatively slower rate of antibody production in vertebrates and suggesting that cell division (see section 4.6) was not involved. Although this factor, once isolated, could be used to transfer protection to non-infected insects, it showed a further distinction from antibody molecules in the fact that it was secreted as promptly after mechanical damage as after exposure to bacterial infection.

Factors with similar properties have been identified in other groups, and in the lobster, for example, a specific memory component has been demonstrated. This more sophisticated response may have evolved from a generalized reaction to physiological trauma in the broad sense. However the actual bases of memory and of the specificity by which bacterial lysis is achieved (but not, presumably, lysis of the host's own cells) remain to be explained.

The invertebrate response which shows the closest relationship to its vertebrate counterpart is that of graft rejection, and the ability to recognize and respond to foreign tissue grafts has proved to be very widespread among the invertebrate phyla, including more lowly groups such as the Coelenterata. It is therefore a phenomenon which is associated, in the evolutionary sense, with the whole history of multicellular life and with the sort of tissue interaction and recognition mechanisms which were discussed earlier. However it should be made clear that graft rejection in the more lowly groups is often a sluggish affair and also that the situation in coelenterates differs from that seen in vertebrates in one important respect; no memory component has yet been demonstrated. On the other hand, rejection responses in earthworms, which have been particularly well studied, result in the rapid destruction of primary grafts when tissue is exchanged between worms of different genera within the family Lumbricidae, and clear evidence of specific memory (Fig. 2–3). The response in worms is less rapid when grafts are exchanged between different individuals within a single species, and the incidence of successful rejection may not exceed 15%. This is in contrast to the situation in man, where intraspecific grafts (heart, kidney or skin transplants) are invariably rejected with great speed unless most careful steps are taken to 'tissue match' donor

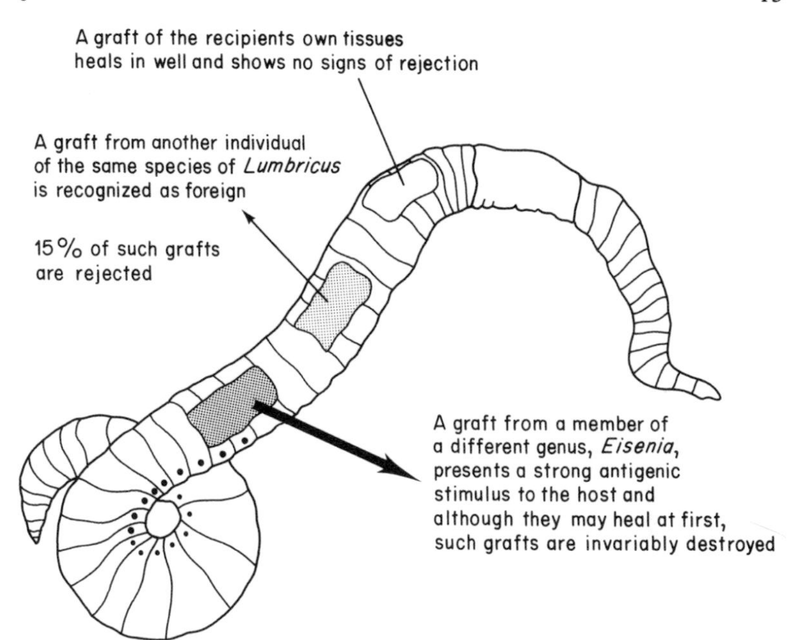

Fig. 2–3 Skin graft rejection in the earthworm *Lumbricus*. Cooper has suggested that antigenic differences between worms of the same genus are few, and that coelomocytes only carry few receptors for these antigens. On the other hand coelomocytes are well provided with receptors to detect the strong antigenic differences which exist between worms of different species. (Data from Cooper, E. L. (1976). '*Comparative Immunology*', J. J. Marchalonis (ed.). Blackwells, Oxford.)

and recipient, and, usually, to subject the recipient to some form of immunosuppressive treatment.

Whether this low rate of rejection within a single earthworm species implies that worm populations are genetically homogeneous, or whether it means that their immune recognition mechanisms are relatively insensitive remains to be determined. Of more importance, perhaps, is the question as to why an earthworm from Oregon should be equipped to reject grafts from its Canadian cousins, since exposure to grafted tissue is unlikely to have numbered among the selective pressures experienced by its annelid ancestors. (This question, of course, is equally pertinent to transplantation responses in vertebrates and is considered in more detail in Chapter 6.)

2.5 Do invertebrates possess lymphocytes?

Among the higher invertebrates graft rejection has been shown to occur not only in the annelids but also in echinoderms and chordates such as the tunicates. In echinoderms as well as annelids memory has also been demonstrated. Surprisingly, perhaps, graft rejection has not been as clearly established for the arthropods where life span, moulting patterns and the efficient encapsulation response combine to make critical experiments difficult to perform. However, cell-mediated immunity is clearly an invertebrate as well as a vertebrate phenomenon, and its demonstration in primitive chordates and echinoderms provides an opportunity for tracing the evolutionary origins of the vertebrate system.

The cells involved in graft rejection in annelids are best described as coelomocytes, and three morphologically distinct families of cell are recognized. Graft rejection is accompanied by cellular invasion of the grafted tissue in a manner which is highly reminiscent of rejection in mammals, and while the invading coelomocytes show phagocytic activity, they also respond by cell division when set up in culture with the non-specific mitogens phytohaemagglutinin and concanavalin A. In vertebrates a mitotic response to these agents is diagnostic for that family of lymphocytes which is responsible for cell-mediated immunity, the T-lymphocytes (see Chapter 4), so there are strong parallels between the situations in earthworms and in vertebrates. On the other hand the very distant evolutionary relationship between the two groups precludes us for the present from describing coelomocytes in vertebrate terms.

In contrast, in protochordates and echinoderms, a series of cells have been described which show close morphological similarity to cells involved in vertebrate immunity. These include cells which Hildemann has described as distinctive lymphocytes, granulocytes and macrophages, and cellular infiltrates associated with graft rejection in echinoderms include representatives of all these types. Furthermore it is an essential characteristic of these primitive immunocompetent cells that they are mobile cells, transported in the body fluids and able to afford defence to all parts of the organism. In these respects cell-mediated immunity in these invertebrate groups has close links with the vertebrate system and may prove to be the foundation from which vertebrate mechanisms evolved. On the other hand there is no evidence for organization of these cells into lympho-reticular tissues such as are found in vertebrates, and from this point of view the Agnatha represent the true beginnings of vertebrate immunity. Whether putative invertebrate lymphocytes deserve that classification really awaits more detailed analysis of their plasma membrane in the light of what we now know about the nature of antigen receptors and other structures on the surface of vertebrate lymphocytes.

3 Antibodies and Antigens

3.1 General properties of antibody molecules

The essential feature which differentiates vertebrate humoral immunity from its invertebrate counterparts is its specificity. This in turn is primarily dependent on antibody molecules whose three-dimensional shape allows each to bind to one particular antigenic determinant. The high degree of specificity which is inherent in the antibody-antigen interaction is not only fundamental to the success of antibodies as a defence mechanism in vertebrates, but is also the basis of many diagnostic tests in biological and medical laboratories. Antibodies are used, for instance, in determining blood group compatibility, in identifying strains of bacteria or viruses during epidemics, and for detecting both the presence and the quantity of many constituents of tissues and body fluids. In the laboratory these reactions may be visualized as the agglutination of particles such as bacteria, or the precipitation of protein antigens, for example in gel (Figs 3–1 and 3–2), although more precise methods using isotopically labelled antigens or antibodies are now often used.

The *in vivo* consequences of the antibody–antigen interaction depend upon the particular identities of the reactants. If the antigen is a virus, combination of antibody with its infective site will inhibit its ability to infect host cells. On the other hand, if the antigen is a product of a bacterial infection, for example tetanus toxin, then interaction with antibody can neutralize the activity of the molecule.

Further effects may follow the initial binding of antibody. As we have seen, antibody-coated molecules or cells are often more easily phagocytosed, while the binding of certain classes of antibody to bacteria will mediate their lysis by activating the components of normal serum known collectively as complement. Thus, in addition to their primary role of binding to antigens, many antibodies have additional properties most of which normally function to improve the defensive capacity of the immune system. These properties are best understood in relation to the molecular structure of the separate antibody classes and are therefore considered in greater detail at a later stage.

Despite the general principle of specificity, antibodies sometimes cross-react with apparently unrelated cells or molecules. In the case of cross-reacting molecules, the effect is usually due to the chance sharing of a particular configuration at the molecular surfaces, or because the molecules are phylogenetically closely related. For example, antibodies

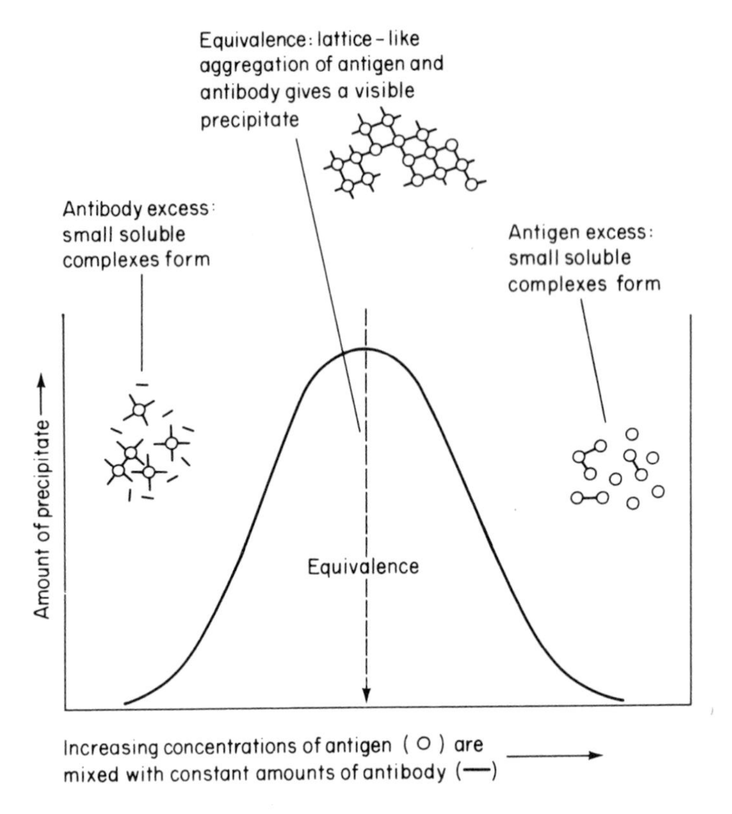

Fig. 3–1 Precipitation of a soluble antigen, such as a protein, with its corresponding antibody. Maximum precipitation is seen only when the reagents are mixed in optimum proportions (i.e. at equivalence) since in antibody or antigen excess soluble complexes tend to be formed.

made in the rabbit against protein components of normal mouse serum react well with several serum proteins from the rat (another myomorph rodent, and therefore a close relative of the mouse), but very much less well with those from the guinea pig (an hystricomorph rodent) or from a more distantly related species.

In the same way, cross reactivity between cells usually occurs because they have identical or closely-related molecules exposed on their surfaces. For example, humans of the blood group O normally have antibodies in their serum which will react with the two blood group antigens A and B. This happens because certain bacteria, living as commensals in the digestive tract, immunize their hosts against bacterial

(a) Ouchterlony assay

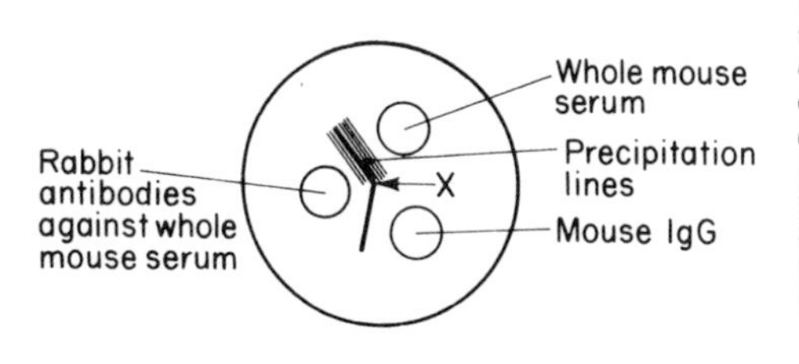

The reagents are placed in wells cut in agar gel in a small plastic dish. They diffuse outwards into the gel, and where antigen and antibody meet in optimal proportions, a visible precipitate forms. The joining of precipitation lines (as at X) indicates the presence of identical antigens

(b) Immunoelectrophoresis

Rabbit antibodies against whole mouse serum

Origin

Gel layered on a glass slide

Albumin IgA IgM IgG

A solution of antigens e.g. whole mouse serum, is placed in a small well, and a current run across the gel to spread the various components of the mixture in a line as shown. When the current is switched off, each component starts to diffuse (arrows) and their presence is detected by addition of appropriate antibody to the centre trough. Many separate components of serum can be revealed in this way. Stage 1 above, stage 2 below

Fig. 3–2 Precipitation of antibodies with antigens in gel is a commonly used technique which is helpful for showing the relationships between different antigens or sets of antigens and for analysing complex mixtures of proteins, such as occurs in mammalian serum. Two techniques are illustrated. Imunoelectrophoresis has the greater sensitivity due to the separation of the antigenic constituents, and clearly distinguishes between different immunoglobulins (Ig) in a serum sample.

cell surface antigens which are identical to the A and B determinants. Individuals of blood group A or B (or both) will not make antibodies to the corresponding bacterial antigen since vertebrates are normally unresponsive towards their own array of antigens (see Chapter 6).

It will be apparent from these examples that the lack of specificity which is observed with cross reactions is more apparent than real. When that particular part of a molecule or cell surface which combines with an antibody is analysed, it is found that the principle of specificity of reaction is upheld.

3.2 Antibody diversity

When a mammal such as a mouse or a rabbit is immunized against a

Table 1 Properties of human antibody (immunoglobulin) classes.

Antibody class	*IgG*	*IgM*	*IgA*	*IgD*	*IgE*
Heavy (H) chains	γ^{a}	μ	α	δ	ε
Light (L) chains	κ or λ	κ or λ	κ or λ	κ or λ	κ or λ
Molecular structure	$\gamma_2 L_2$	$(\mu_2 L_2)_5$	$\alpha_2 L_2{}^{b}$	$\delta_2 L_2$	$\varepsilon_2 L_2$
Molecular weight	150 000	900 000	160 000	180 000	200 000
% carbohydrate	3	12	7	13	11
Additional protein chains	—	J chain	J chain; secretory component [b]	—	—
Serum concentration (mg 100 ml^{-1})	700–1500	60–170	150–400	3.0	0.01–0.03
Antigen-binding sites	2	5 (10)	2	?	2
Functions	Fixes complement; cytophilic for macrophages; crosses placenta[c]	Produced early in antibody response; fixes complement; efficient agglutinin and lysin	Predominant in bodily secretions, protecting against infection via eyes, naso-pharynx, etc.	Receptor (with IgM or IgG) on lymphocyte surface	Binds to mast cells in the tissues; responsible for allergies such as hay fever

a Four subclasses of IgG, each with a distinctive H chain, occur in both man and mouse.
b. IgA is frequently found in the serum as a dimer of structure $[(\alpha_2 L_2)_2 + J]$. Secreted IgA consists of this dimer plus the secretory component, a glycoprotein which ensures its safe passage across tissue barriers into the secretions.
c. Not all subclasses of IgG possess these properties. For instance, human IgG_4 does not fix complement.

foreign protein, it is usually found that the antibodies which are produced vary with respect to molecular weight and to certain other properties, although they all bind to that particular antigen. In fact, five major antibody *classes* have been identified in mammals (Table 1) and each of these has a distinct molecular structure which is class-specific and yet shows clear relationships to that of the remaining classes. Antibodies may be visualized, therefore, as a close-knit yet heterogeneous family of multi-chain proteins, all of which are variations on the same theme.

Because mammals are continually exposed to antigens in the normal course of events, antibodies are found in the serum of all healthy individuals and they may be detected by a variety of means. When serum proteins are fractionated according to their electrophoretic mobility, antibodies are found to be located mainly in the γ-globulin fraction. They are often referred to as *immunoglobulins* (Ig for short).

3.3 Antibody structure

Of the mammalian classes of immunoglobulin IgG is structurally the best understood. A number of basic techniques have been used to determine antibody structure. These include (*i*) reduction and alkylation so as to split intra-molecular disulphide bonds, (*ii*) enzymatic digestion, dividing the molecule into fragments whose separate properties can be identified, (*iii*) amino-acid sequencing of isolated polypeptide chains, and (*iv*) X-ray crystallography. The last two of these techniques in particular have been greatly helped by the increasing availability in recent years of both human and rodent lymphocyte tumour (myeloma) cell lines which produce large quantities of homogeneous antibodies. These are often better suited to study than the mixture of antibodies which is found in normal serum.

Much of our understanding of antibody structure is based on the Nobel Prize-winning work of R. R. Porter in England and G. M. Edelman in the United States, as a result of which Porter made the proposal that IgG is composed of four polypeptide chains linked together by disulphide bonds (Fig. 3–3). It was shown that when IgG molecules are broken down to their component chains by reduction and alkylation, two types of chain can be identified. The larger, or 'heavy', chain has a molecular weight of about 50 000 daltons, and is composed of some 450 amino acids, while the smaller 'light' chain, with about 220 amino acids, has a molecular weight around 23 000 daltons. The exact figures vary between species and between IgG subclasses.

Each IgG molecule consists of two heavy (H) and two light (L) chains. When the chains are separated and tested for their individual ability to bind antigen, isolated H chains show some binding activity and isolated L chains show little or none. This suggests that the antigen-binding sites

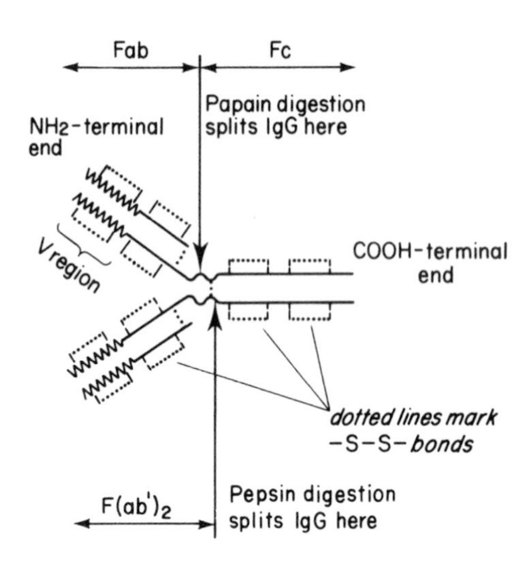

Fig. 3–3 Diagram of an IgG molecule to show arrangement of heavy and light chains with V regions (ᴡᴡᴡᴡ) and disulphide bonds (dotted lines). Sites of pepsin and papain cleavage are also shown (redrawn after FUDENBERG H. H. *et al.*, 1978).

of IgG depend in some way upon the interaction of the component chains, a conclusion which is supported by evidence from other experimental approaches. For instance, a strong indication that the binding sites for antigen are located at the NH_2-terminal end of each H–L pair is provided by studies on enzymatic digestion of the whole molecule. It was first shown by Porter that papain treatment splits the IgG molecule into three fragments, two of which are identical and consist of a whole L chain plus the NH_2-terminal half of one H chain (Fig. 3–3). These two fragments contain all the antigen-binding activity of the whole molecule and they were subsequently termed the Fab pieces (Fragment antigen-binding). The third fragment consists only of the COOH-terminal halves of the two H chains, joined by disulphide bonds, and has no antigen-binding activity. It was termed the Fc piece (Fragment crystallizable) since it could be crystallized out of solution with relative ease.

Similar studies by Edelman, using pepsin to cleave the IgG molecule, supported Porter's findings. Pepsin treatment produces a single large fragment and many small polypeptide chains. The large fragment contains all the antigen-binding activity and on reduction and alkylation it splits into two identical pieces, each slightly larger than Fab. The large fragment is thus known as $F(ab')_2$ (Fig. 3–3).

Electron microscope and other studies have shown that the region near the inter-H chain disulphide bonds is flexible and should be regarded as a hinge region which permits variable positioning of the binding sites relative to each other. The molecular basis for the position and the specificity of the two IgG binding sites has become clear as a result of amino-acid sequencing studies from which the complete sequence of many isolated chains and some whole immunoglobulins are now known.

Comparisons made between the amino-acid sequences of different chains show that both H and L chains can be divided into *constant* and *variable* regions. The constant region is that in which there is a high degree of similarity in the arrangement of amino acids in most immunoglobulins studied. The variable regions, on the other hand, are characterized by distinct sections where the sequences are unique to immunoglobulins of any one specificity, resulting, for each antibody, in an unique three dimensional shape. In this way the antigen-binding site of each antibody is formed. Each binding site, determined in this way, can also act as an antigenic determinant against which antibodies may be made. These determinants must also be unique for immunoglobulins of a single specificity and are known as *idiotypes*.

The variable (V) region occupies the NH_2-terminal half of each L chain and the NH_2-terminal quarter of each H chain. The constant (C) region occupies the remainder of each chain, although the exact point where the V-region ends and the C-region begins varies from class to class of antibody and from species to species of animal.

With the exception of certain residues, particularly cysteine, which are important for the tertiary structure of each chain, it is usual to find one of from two to five 'possible' amino acids occurring at each point in the variable region. At certain portions of the variable region, however, *hypervariable* sequences have been identified in which virtually all positions are variable and in which some positions may be occupied by any of several (usually more than five) amino acids. Three such hypervariable spots have been identified in L chains, and three or four in H chains, depending on the species.

In order to understand the significance of the hypervariable regions, it is first necessary to consider another aspect of H and L chain structure, namely the distribution of intra-chain disulphide bonds. There are two such links within each L chain and four in each H chain and their effect is to throw the chains into loops of approximately equal size (Fig. 3–4). In 1971, Edelman proposed that each loop with its adjacent portions of chain should be regarded as a 'domain', endowed with a specific function. The C-region domains in both L and H chains are connected with various secondary properties of the immunoglobulin molecule, but the V-region domains (V_L and V_H) have the function of forming the antigen-

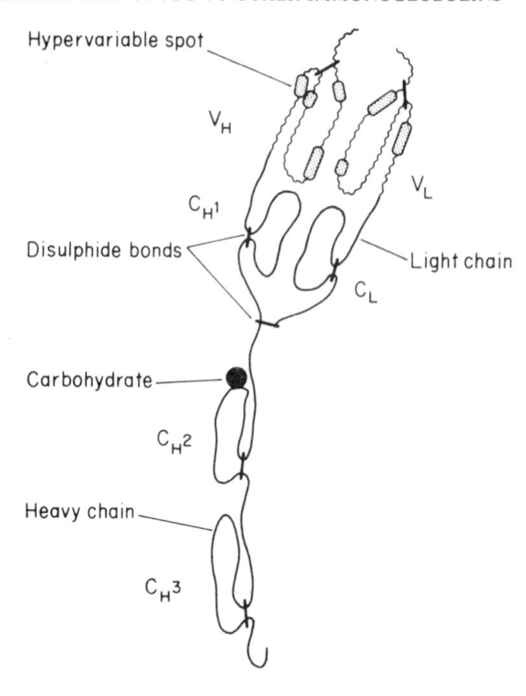

Fig. 3–4 Diagram to illustrate the folding of heavy and light chains due to the presence of intrachain disulphide bonds, and the position of the various domains. Within the variable regions (~~~~~~), the positions of hypervariable spots are shown (shaded areas). One half only of an IgG molecule is represented.

binding sites. It is found that the hypervariable spots are situated in, or closely adjacent to, the V_L and V_H loops (Fig. 3–4). The technique of affinity labelling, whereby a radioactive molecule is chemically transferred from an antigen to that part of the antibody molecule with which it binds, confirms the importance of the hypervariable regions for the antigen-binding site. After dissociation of antigen and antibody, the label is found to be associated with the hypervariable spots.

3.4 The relationship of IgG to the other immunoglobulin classes

It has already been stated that there are fundamental similarities between the major classes of mammalian immunoglobulin (Fig. 3–5). In fact all five are based on the four polypeptide chain model (2H + 2L) described for IgG and differ from each other primarily in that each class has a unique H chain structure, and also in that two of the classes, IgM

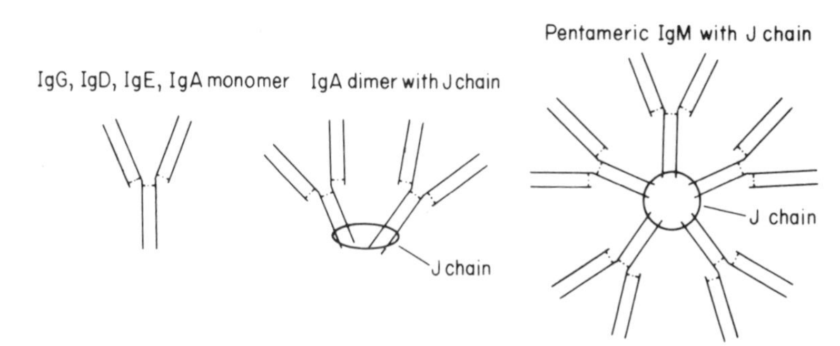

Fig. 3–5 The structural relationships of the immunoglobulin classes. Mammalian IgM, a pentamer, has a potential 10 binding sites for antigen, but in practice only 5 can be occupied. In lower vertebrates, tetrameric and hexameric IgMs occur. In both IgM and IgA the J chain is attached within the antibody synthesizing cell (otherwise molecules of mixed specificity would be found). The position of the disulphide bonds joining H chains or linking H to L is variable depending on species, antibody class and, where these occur, subclass. Secretory IgA is characterized by the inclusion of an additional glycoprotein molecule, the secretory piece.

and IgA, exist as polymers of the basic structure, in association with additional polypeptide chains. There are also functional differences between the classes which are described in the next section.

The differences in H chain structure reside both in amino-acid sequences and in associated carbohydrate, and the distinct H chains are named μ, γ, α, δ and ε after the molecule (IgM, G, A, D, E) in which they are found (see Table 1). In addition, the IgG class in particular is further subdivided into subclasses, also on the basis of H chain structure and functional differences. There are four subclasses in man, and up to four have been described for different species of rodent.

L chains do not differ between classes of immunoglobulin. However, two types of L chain have been described, and these are known as kappa (κ) and lambda (λ). Both κ and λ chains may be associated with any immunoglobulin class, but in a single antibody molecule both (or all) L chains are of the same type. Both types are normally found in any one individual, but the balance of the two varies from species to species. In primates and rodents, for example, most immunoglobulin molecules have the κ chain while the λ chain predominates in carnivores, ungulates and birds. Comparison of amino-acid sequences between the C_κ and C_λ regions of man or mouse shows 35–40% homology between them and suggests that κ and λ have a common evolutionary origin. However, mouse C_κ and human C_κ show still greater homology, as also do mouse C_λ and human C_λ, indicating that the κ–λ divergence occurred before the ancestral lines of mouse and man separated. There is some evidence that it may have occurred much earlier, among the fishes. Presumably, there are strong selective forces maintaining κ and λ as distinct co-existent chains, although no clear demarcation of function has been found between them.

3.5 Functional characteristics of immunoglobulin classes

Most of the serum immunoglobulin of normal placental mammals is IgG. IgM, however, has a longer evolutionary history, stretching back to primitive fishes. The evolutionary development of IgG and other Ig classes is less clear than for IgM. Molecules which are distinct from IgM appear in the lungfishes and then in amphibians, reptiles and birds, but their relationship to mammalian IgG is uncertain.

Following primary immunization of a mammal such as a rat or mouse the first specific antibody molecules to appear are IgM, and their multiple binding sites make them very efficient in dealing with multivalent antigens such as viruses or bacteria. Because of their size, IgM molecules are mostly retained within the blood vascular system, and they are therefore of particular importance in systemic infections.

Subsequently, IgM is replaced by IgG which is the predominant antibody in late primary and in secondary responses. (Exceptions are responses to certain antigens, particularly polysaccharides, which do not involve T cell 'help' (see Chapter 5); in these, little or no IgG antibody is produced.) On account of its smaller size IgG has a wider distribution among the tissue fluids, and it is also unique in being able to cross the placenta from mother to foetus and thus afford protection to the developing mammal. This may be an important evolutionary step in the development of viviparity.

One function of IgG is the inactivation of bacterial toxins, and the neutralization of viruses by binding to their active sites, but the additional properties of the molecule allow it to play a wider role in defence. For example, IgG antibodies can act as opsonins, promoting the phagocytosis and digestion of bacteria, by virtue of the presence, on the Fc portion of the molecule, of a binding site for the cell membrane of macrophages and blood monocytes (Fig. 2–2). Although antibody-coated bacteria, for instance, are more rapidly phagocytosed as a result of this mechanism, attachment to antigen is not an essential prerequisite for binding of IgG to macrophage membranes.

A further property of some IgG subclasses, as well as IgM, is their ability to initiate the sequential activation of a series of serum proteins known collectively as '*complement*'. Activation results in the lysis of cellular antigens such as bacteria, together with other effects including

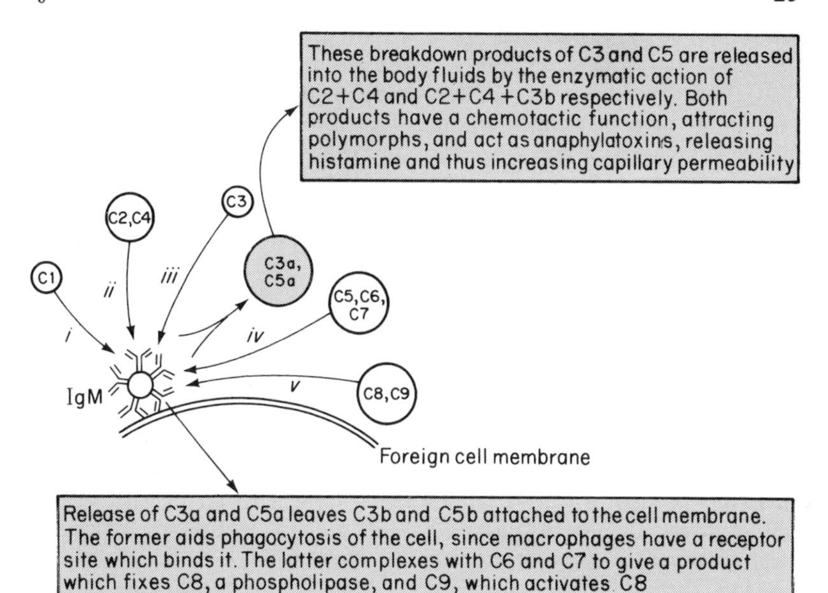

Fig. 3–6 The classical pathway of complement fixation, initiated by the binding of C1q to two adjacent Fc pieces (in this case in a single IgM molecule). C1r and C1s follow, and then the sequence is as shown. Eventually C8 and C9 provide the cytolytic activity. Note the way in which products of C3 and C5 involve phagocytic cells. The central event in the whole sequence is the fixation and splitting of C3, and this may also be achieved by the so-called 'alternate pathway' in which an alternative C3 convertase is activated, independently of the presence of antibody, by the influence of a variety of extrinsic substances, notably bacterial polysaccharides.

the chemotactic attraction of phagocytic cells to the site of infection (Fig. 3–6). The activation of complement is associated with the antibody Fc region, but only occurs after antigen has been bound at the NH_2-terminal end; presumably some structural alteration exposes the complement-activating site. In man, the IgG subclasses 1, 2 and 3 activate complement, but the most efficient activation in man and other mammals is achieved by IgM. This is because the initial step is the binding of the first component of complement (C1q) to two adjacent Fc sites. With IgM these are provided on the same molecule, and therefore only one molecule of IgM is required to initiate lysis of an antigenic cell whereas, with IgG, two separate molecules must bind in close proximity on the antigen's surface before C1q will be fixed.

The association of these additional properties with the Fc region of antibody proteins has led Edelman to propose that the antibody molecule is so organized that each domain has a specific function (Fig. 3–4). Those in the V-region of the two polypeptide chains (called V_H and V_L) are involved in antigen binding. The two COOH-terminal domains of the H chain (C_{H^2} and C_{H^3}) are associated with complement fixation and macrophage binding respectively, but no function has yet been ascribed to the remaining two domains (C_L and C_{H^1}).

3.6 Antigens

Antigens are those substances which bind to lymphocyte receptors and initiate an immune response. Many cells, including bacteria and foreign erythrocytes, are antigenic in mammals and other vertebrates, and may provoke vigorous antibody production. Detailed analysis shows that the antigenicity of cells such as these depends upon the molecular constitution of their cell membranes. For example, the A and B blood groups in man are determined by cell surface carbohydrate molecules, while the H antigens which are diagnostic for different strains and species of *Salmonella* are flagellar proteins.

Only the biological macromolecules – proteins, carbohydrates and perhaps, to a limited extent, nucleic acids–are truly antigenic; smaller molecules and, usually, nucleic acids are only antigenic when bound to proteins. The physical properties of each species of macromolecule are important in determining the degree of antigenicity, and chief among these is the requirement for size. It is not easy, for example, to make antibodies against insulin, a protein of 10 000 daltons, while proteins of less than 4–5000 daltons are only rarely antigenic. The minimum antigenic size for polysaccharides is considerably greater.

If one takes even a smallish antigen, say a protein like insulin, and examines its interaction with antibody, it is found that only a small part of the antigenic molecule actually fits into the antibody-binding site. That is to say, antibodies, and therefore presumably lymphocyte receptors, do not recognize the whole antigen at one time, but only parts of it, the so-called *antigenic determinants* or *epitopes*. Studies on the inhibition of antibody–antigen interactions by the use of antigen fragments have shown that the antibody binding site can accommodate a molecular fragment of up to 1000 daltons (Fig. 3–7), although in many cases it is clear that the determinant size is less than this. Thus, a protein antigen should be regarded as a molecule whose surface is a network of potential determinant sites, which may physically overlap each other so that points on the molecular surface may contribute to more than one epitope. Antigenic determinants are defined in strictly functional terms in that they can only be identified if some sort of reaction is initiated against them. It is largely a matter of chance how many facets of a

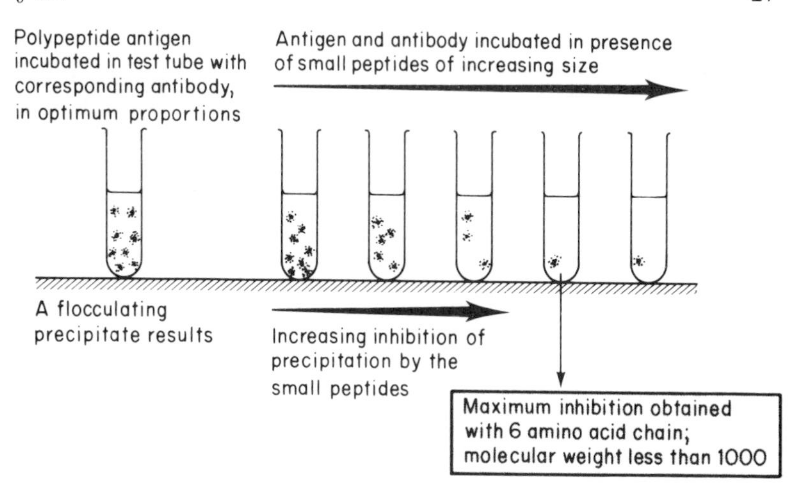

Fig. 3–7 Demonstration of inhibition of precipitation of an antigen by low molecular weight polypeptides, obtained by digestion of the antigen.

protein's surface are recognized by lymphocyte receptors during the course of an immune response.

3.7 Carriers and haptens

There is an obvious paradox in the story outlined in the previous section, in that we have defined the functional antigenic determinant as being relatively small, while we have also stated that molecules are better antigens if they are large. This has led, particularly in the context of antibody responses to proteins which depend on help from T-lymphocytes, to the division of antigenic molecules into two parts, the epitope or determinant, and the bulk of the molecule – the *carrier*. In the response to any one determinant, it has been postulated that B-lymphocytes are stimulated by that determinant, while 'helper' T-lymphocytes respond to the carrier. This view of the antigenic molecule has considerable implications for our understanding of cell interactions during immune responses (see Chapter 5), but it must be appreciated at this stage that the part of an antigen which is defined as 'carrier' for one particular epitope may itself include determinants which can stimulate B-lymphocytes in their own right.

The experimental requirements of much recent immunology have led to the use of artificial antigens in which small molecules, not antigenic on their own but whose chemical composition is precisely known, have been bound to an appropriate protein or carbohydrate carrier (the term 'carrier' derives from these sorts of experiment). In this way it has been possible to investigate responses to single defined determinants (often called *haptens*) by, for example, measuring the reaction of the antibodies with the same hapten bound to another carrier. Our understanding of antibody structure and heterogeneity, and of lymphocyte receptors has been greatly increased by such techniques.

4 Lymphoid Cells and Tissues

The primary function of lymphocytes is to recognize the presence of anything alien in the body: this they do with a precision unmatched in any other group of animals. They thus have a central role in what is undoubtedly one of the most important and pervasive features of vertebrate physiology. Twenty years ago, it was still possible to speak of 'the lymphocyte'. Despite its widespread distribution, it seemed a small uninteresting-looking cell with little cytoplasm, and its function was unclear. Since then, however, it has become evident that the term 'lymphocyte' really encompasses a family of cells, each member of which plays a distinct role in the immune system. All these cells have much the same unremarkable appearance in the light or electron microscope, but they differ in ontogeny and lifespan and when stimulated by antigen differentiate into effector cells according to their particular function. The most fundamental division in the lymphocyte family is between B-(bursa-derived) and T-(thymus-derived) lymphocytes, but it has now become clear that T-cells in particular may be further subdivided into several distinct populations.

4.1 Lymphocyte diversity

B-lymphocytes are the precursors of plasma cells whose function is to manufacture and secrete antibodies. Each B-cell is equipped with receptors for antigen which are, in fact, antibody molecules, synthesized by the lymphocyte, and expressed on its surface. Under the right circumstances, binding of antigen to these receptors initiates a series of mitotic divisions accompanied by differentiation to plasma cells and to modified B-lymphocytes known as 'memory' cells. The memory cells constitute an expanded population of lymphocytes which can react against the particular antigen concerned, and they help to ensure that if the animal is re-exposed to the same antigen, a rapid antibody response will ensue. Since each lymphocyte is pre-committed to make molecules of just one antibody specificity, the surface receptors are identical in specificity and affinity to the antibody molecules which are formed and secreted by the descendant plasma cells.

The functions of T-lymphocytes are more complex and more varied. Firstly, they act as regulators of the activity of B-lymphocytes with the capacity either to enhance or to suppress antibody synthesis. In addition, certain of them can be stimulated by grafts of foreign tissue, or by virus-infected cells, to differentiate into 'killer' T-lymphocytes which can specifically kill the foreign or virus-carrying cells. Finally, they can recruit macrophages as effector cells, as in graft rejection and certain kinds of allergic reaction.

Like B-lymphocytes, T-cells are initially activated by the combination of an antigen with antigen-specific receptors on the cell surface, although these receptors are probably not immunoglobulin molecules. Again, population expansion follows together with the generation of memory and effector cells, but there the resemblance ends; no plasma cells are produced and, apart from the killer cells, the effectors act indirectly through their influence on B-cells, macrophages and possibly other cells. The ways in which they do this are discussed in Chapters 5 and 6.

Besides their functional differences B- and T-lymphocytes may also be distinguished on the basis of unique cell surface molecules which have been identified either because they have a specific immunological function, or because they are antigenic and will bind specific antibodies. These surface markers may be used not only to distinguish lymphocytes, but also to separate them into populations which are greatly enriched for one class or the other (see section 7.3).

In the mouse the most widely used marker for T-lymphocytes is the Thy 1 alloantigen, originally known as 'theta'. Two alleles have been recognized in inbred mouse strains, resulting in the expression of Thy 1.1 or Thy 1.2, depending on the strain. Antibody prepared against this antigen will lyse Thy 1-bearing cells in the presence of the complement components of normal serum, thus enriching a lymphocyte population for Thy 1 negative cells (in effect, B-lymphocytes). Alternatively, if a fluorescent antibody is used and complement is excluded, the proportion of Thy 1 positive cells can be estimated. In addition to Thy 1, mouse T-lymphocytes also carry markers belonging to two series of membrane components, the Lyt and Qat differentiation antigens. It has been found that Lyt 1, 2 and 3 occur in different combinations on T-lymphocyte surfaces, and these can be used to identify functional subpopulations of this cell class.

B-lymphocytes also have markers, of which the presence of readily detectable surface immunoglobulin, in the form of receptors for antigen, is the most characteristic. Most B-cells also carry Ia antigens (see section 6.2), and surface receptors for the Fc part of Ig molecules and for the third component of complement. B-cell specific differentiation antigens, analogous to the Lyt set on T-cells, have also been described recently and these may prove to have interesting correlations with B-cell function.

4.2 Ontogeny of lymphocytes

Lymphocytes are descended, via one of at least two differentiation pathways, from pluripotent haematopoietic stem cells which are found, for instance, in mammalian bone marrow. 'Pluripotent' implies that the stem cells, besides reproducing themselves, can differentiate into all the cellular elements of blood: erythrocytes, granulocytes, monocytes and platelets, as well as lymphocytes. The main steps as they occur in the mouse, and probably other mammals, are shown in Fig. 4–1.

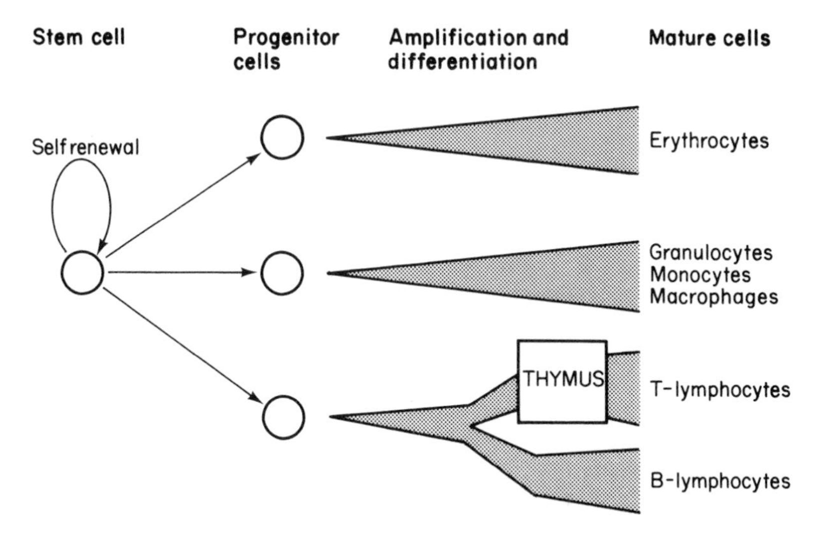

Fig. 4–1 Differentiation pathways of lymphocytes and some other blood elements in mammals. In the adult, most stages take place within the bone marrow, although T-lymphocyte differentiation proceeds in the thymus gland. The spleen is also an important source of haematopoiesis, as is the liver in embryonic life. Progenitor cells in the marrow share with multipotent stem cells the capacity to self renew.

4.2.1 T-lymphocytes

The differentiation pathway for T-lymphocytes includes a period of residence and proliferation in the thymus gland. The thymus is basically an epithelial organ, and contact of the developing T-lymphocytes with epithelial cells seems to be important in helping them to learn the distinction between 'self' and 'not-self' and hence in avoiding destructive autoimmune reactions. The thymus also produces certain chemical factors for which various functional claims have been made. Some of these, including a pentapeptide called thymopoietin, have been purified. Thymopoietin, and possibly other factors, may supplement or to some extent substitute for the micro-environmental influence of the intact thymus. It must be emphasized that some features of the differentiation and maturation of T- (and B-) lymphocytes remain poorly understood. In particular, there is a shadowy area between the haematopoietic stem cell and the lymphocytes of the thymus. When and where does a stem cell become committed to producing T-cells and nothing but T-cells? Can these 'committed' progenitors reproduce themselves as well as differentiate, (that is, are they truly lymphoid 'stem cells') or do they need constant replenishment from the pluripotent stem cell compartment? Is there an intermediate stage at which a cell becomes committed to producing T- *and* B-lymphocyte descendants, before the T *versus* B decision is made? To these questions definitive answers are still lacking.

4.2.2 B-lymphocytes

B-lymphocytes are produced more or less fully-fledged from mammalian bone marrow (B for bone marrow, as it happens, although strictly speaking B stands for the bursa of Fabricius, a specialized lympho-epithelial organ which provides the essential microenvironment for B-cell differentiation in birds, but which is absent in mammals). A B-lymphocyte may be said to be recognizable as such when it starts to manufacture immunoglobulin (Ig). In the foetal mouse, cells with intracytoplasmic Ig can first be seen in the liver on the 12th day of gestation (total gestation period = 20 days), and Ig may be found on the surface by the 16th day. The Ig at this stage consists exclusively of 'monomeric' fragments of IgM (that is, two L-chains and two μ-chains). In the late foetus and neonate the focus of B-cell formation shifts to the spleen, and in the adult to the bone marrow. Adult mouse marrow exports 10^7–10^8 young B-cells per day, mainly to the spleen. As maturation proceeds, other classes of Ig may be found on the surface of B-cells. One such is IgD, which seems not to be present until several days after birth. Thereafter many B-cells carry both IgM and IgD on their surface. Since the specificity of each molecule for antigen is apparently identical, it is not obvious why there should be two types of receptor molecule. One suggestion is that both molecules are needed to transfer the necessary differentiative signals to the interior of the cell when the appropriate antigen is encountered; in the absence of IgD, the cell may be inactivated or rendered 'tolerant' (see Chapter 6), and the presence of an 'IgM only' stage in B-cell maturation may be important in developing necessary tolerance to self antigens. Relatively few B-cells have been shown to carry IgG, A or E on their surface. Some recent evidence suggests that IgG, at least, only appears after antigenic stimulation and is typical of memory cells which will, if re-exposed to antigen, give rise to

IgG-secreting plasma cells. IgG-carrying cells may or may not also carry IgD, and there is some suggestion of a maturation sequence, IgD being lost in the later stages. However, as techniques for detecting cell surface Igs become sharpened and refined, it may well turn out that molecules now believed to be absent from a cell are in fact present in small quantities.

4.3 Generation of diversity

Lymphocytes are perhaps the most individual of cells: each carries its own peculiar specificity for a particular antigenic determinant. Apart from those clones which are expanded as a consequence of exposure to antigen, there will be very few lymphocytes of identical specificity in the body at any time – possibly no more than one. It follows that during ontogeny the lymphocyte population somehow becomes greatly diversified with respect to antigen recognition, but the way in which this happens is still not entirely clear. The two extreme possibilities which have been canvassed are (*i*) that the genome contains information for thousands of different H and L polypeptide chains – identical as far as the constant region goes, but variable at the NH_2-terminal end – and that only one set is expressed in a given cell; and (*ii*) that there is but one germ-line gene for each class (κ, λ, μ, α, etc.) of chain, the diversity being generated anew in each individual animal by somatic mutation. For many reasons, neither of these mechanisms looks at all plausible. Very recently, molecular biologists have begun to accept that pieces of DNA may be shuffled around and spliced onto other pieces. It is indeed already clear that genes coding for the V-region and C-region of an immunoglobulin polypeptide chain can exist separately and become joined together. It also appears increasingly likely that smaller lengths of DNA, coding for the hypervariable regions which determine antibody specificity, can be inserted into the framework of a relatively small number of V-region genes. However it happens, the important point to remember is that diversity is generated, building up repertoires of perhaps 10^7 or more specificities. Subsequently, when an antigen enters the system, it will bind to and activate those lymphocytes carrying complementary receptors. Since each activated cell multiplies up into a clone of daughter cells, this process has been termed 'clonal selection'.

It seems virtually certain that diversity is generated separately in B- and T-lymphocyte populations, since the two differentiate in separate anatomical sites. However, since T-cell receptors carry at least some of the same idiotypic specificities as do immunoglobulins, the genetic blueprints, consisting of DNA for the hypervariable segments, and possibly the whole heavy-chain variable region, are probably the same, even though the complete T-cell receptor is not recognizable as an immunoglobulin.

4.4 Evolution of lymphoid cells and tissues

We have already mentioned that, for the time being at least, lymphocytes should be regarded as being confined to the vertebrates. Similarly, the specific tissues which make and accommodate lymphocytes also have their origin within the vertebrate subphylum. The evolution of major groups is depicted in Fig. 4–2, along with the occurrence of various immunological cells, tissues and functions. Obviously, we can only ascertain the presence of a given function or a particular tissue in animals that are alive today: about their ancestors, we can only speculate. Thus, the fact that lymphocytes and antibodies are

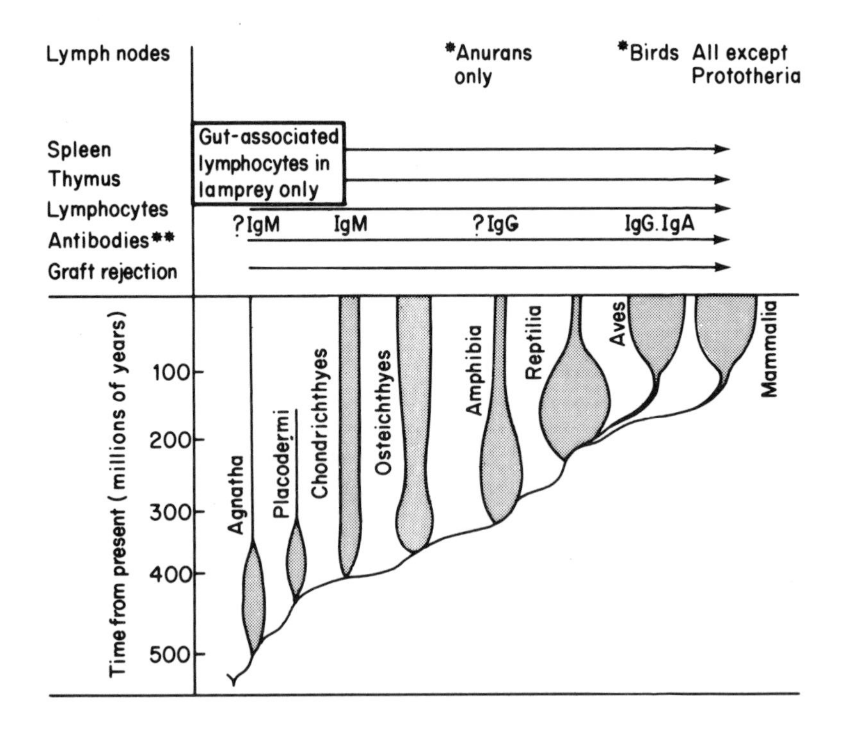

* In anurans and birds clusters of lymphocytes are found in lymphatic vessels, but not true lymph nodes, these being confined to higher mammals

** First appearances of antibodies of various classes are indicated. Low molecular weight antibodies are found in fish but they seem more closely related to monomeric IgM than to IgG.

Fig. 4–2 Evolution of the vertebrates and the development of vertebrate immunity.

present in lampreys as well as mammals does not prove them to have evolved in the early Palaeozoic. It does quite strongly suggest such a thing, but there are enough examples of parallel evolution to make one wary of uncritical acceptance. Such caution is certainly justified when considering the possible homologues in cyclostomes of the mammalian thymus and spleen. Larval lampreys have foci of lymphocytes, in the region of the gills, and these could well be homologous with the thymus which, in land vertebrates, is formed embryologically from branchial epithelium. On the other hand, hagfish lack these aggregates. Cartilaginous fishes have a thymus in which cortex and medulla are already distinct, and all higher vertebrates appear to possess the organ at least when young. The lamprey also has a possible homologue of the spleen, in the form of an aggregate of lymphocytes associated with the anterior part of the gut. Again, cartilaginous fishes and all higher vertebrates possess spleens in which red and white pulps (see section 4.5) are distinguishable.

Lymph nodes, in contrast, are relatively recent evolutionary innovations, found in a fully developed form only in marsupials and placental mammals. The most primitive mammals, the Prototheria, exemplified by the spiny anteater *Echidna*, do not have any proper nodes, but only small nodules within the main lymphatic vessels. Evolution seems to have made more than one attempt to produce lymph node-like structures, since anuran amphibians possess clusters of lymphocytes in some lymphatic vessels, while urodeles, which are considered to be less specialized and closer to the mainstream of vertebrate evolution, do not. Lymph nodes are highly organized structures, well endowed with both lymphocytes and phagocytes, and adapted to provide a controlled response to antigenic stimulation. They are also the major point at which lymphocytes leave the blood, passing via the tissues to the lymphatic circulation, and their vasculature is specially adapted for this purpose. Lymph nodes are often found in strategic locations towards the periphery of the body where they act as an outer defence against local infections. Related structures, the Peyer's patches, are associated with the wall of the small intestine, a further source of possible infection.

The avian bursa of Fabricius is of particular interest, since it is the one discrete organ in any group of animals which is concerned with the primary production of B-lymphocytes. Indeed, the almost complete separation of function between thymus-derived and bursa-derived lymphocytes in the chicken provided the original means of drawing the T *versus* B distinction. Early removal of the thymus from both birds and mammals results in a deficit of cell-mediated immunity, but only in birds can immunoglobulin synthesis be suppressed by a surgical operation, bursectomy. The bursa, a pouch off the cloaca, resembles the thymus in having an epithelial framework which becomes populated with lymphocytes early in ontogeny. The T *versus* B distinction has turned out to be as clear-cut in mammals as in birds, but the micro-environment for B differentiation is, as detailed earlier, more diffuse.

4.5 Functional organization of lymphoid tissues

4.5.1 Lymphocyte traffic

The lymphocytes which occupy the mammalian spleen and lymph nodes are acquired from the blood stream, but their traffic from the blood is a carefully regulated affair. Routes of entry and exit are precisely laid down, and rates of entry may be varied according to changing circumstances.

In the lymph nodes, entry of lymphocytes is across the endothelium of the small post-capillary venules in the cortex. Lymphocytes are able to 'recognize' this particular location, apparently by virtue of recognition molecules on their surface which bind to complementary sites on the endothelial cells. Once bound, the lymphocytes migrate between the endothelial cells and into the tissue of the node (Fig. 4–3), and it has been estimated that around 10–15% of all lymphocytes passing through a lymph node in the blood are diverted into the tissue in this way.

Of the lymphocytes which enter a lymph node, many are destined to have only a short stay, and they will leave within a few hours. They do not return directly to the blood stream, however, but indirectly, via the lymphatic circulation.

All lymph nodes are connected to the lymphatic system, and are provided with afferent and efferent lymphatic ducts. The former bring the watery lymph fluid from the tissues of the body, particularly the skin and the alimentary tract, while the latter drains from the medullary region of the node (Fig. 4–3) and conveys both lymph and migrating lymphocytes back to the blood stream. In some parts of the body the lymph nodes are arranged in chains, and thus the efferent lymphatic of one node becomes the afferent vessel of the next. It is via the afferent lymphatic vessels that antigen is borne to the lymph nodes to initiate an immune response, but the lymph which is collected from the tissues is largely free of cells.

The spleen does not possess the afferent and efferent lymphatic vessels, or the specialized post-capillary venules, of lymph nodes, so that lymphocyte traffic in this organ necessarily follows a different route. Flow is from the blood, via the central arterioles and their branches, to the macrophage-rich marginal zones and thence to discrete lymphoid areas sometimes called the white pulp. Here they take up temporary residence before passing to the red pulp and returning to the bloodstream.

Lymphocytes are thus characteristically a population of cells on the

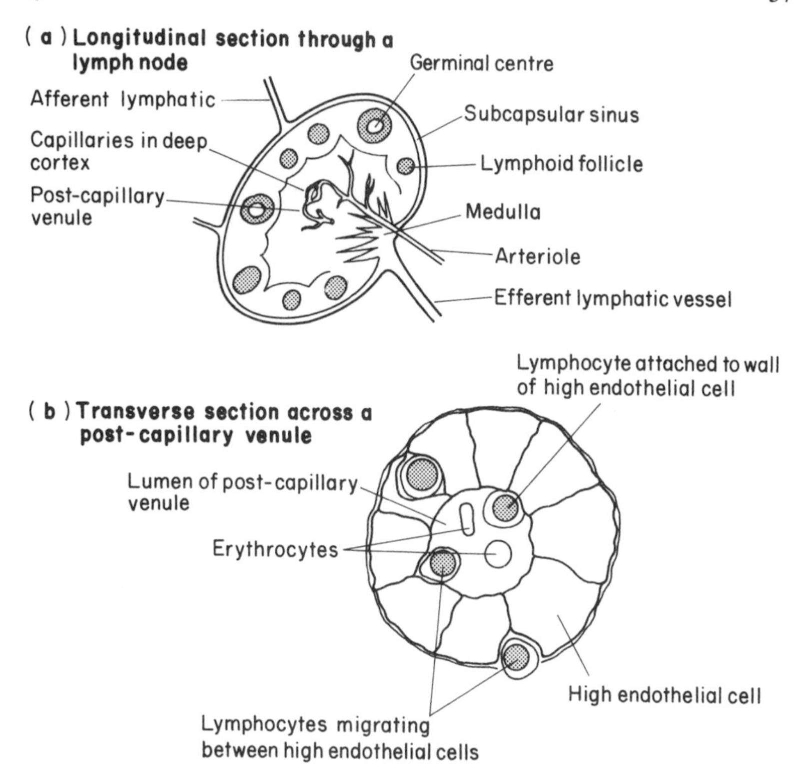

Fig. 4–3 Migration of lymphocytes from blood to lymph. Lymphocytes pass into lymph nodes at the post-capillary venules in the deep cortex. They leave via the efferent lymphatic vessel and are eventually returned to the blood stream via vessels such as the thoracic duct.

move, although for one reason or another, some remain for quite long periods of time within a given tissue. In rodents, the recirculating population travels around the body in a mean time of about 24 hours for B-lymphocytes, slightly less for T-lymphocytes. This process of re-circulation has been shown to be essential for the proper development of immune responses, since the magnitude of a given response is governed more by the flow of cells into an organ than by the number of lymphocytes actually in residence. Two clear advantages of recirculation come to mind; firstly lymphocytes of all specificities (remember, there may only be a few of each) are made available to all parts of the body; secondly, memory cells, once generated at a particular site, perhaps as the result of a clinical immunization, will be disseminated to all parts of the body and provide body-wide protection against subsequent re-infection.

4.5.2 Segregation of lymphocytes in lymphoid organs

The interaction of lymphocytes with other cells mentioned above takes on a new dimension if the distribution of lymphocytes within the lymph nodes and spleen is examined. It is found that T- and B-lymphocytes sort themselves out into discrete areas which remain largely the preserve of either class, even if their number is depleted so as to leave room for immigration by the other type of cell.

In lymph nodes the tissue can be divided into cortex and medulla, the latter being adjacent to the efferent lymphatic duct, and rich in macrophages and migrating lymphocytes. Plasma cells are also found there. The cortex is clearly divided into an outer 'B-dependent' area, characterized particularly by dense clusters of B-lymphocytes known as lymphoid follicles, and an inner 'T-dependent' paracortex in which few B-cells are found (Fig. 4–4). Similarly in the spleen, a cross-section through the white pulp reveals a central arteriole around which is a core

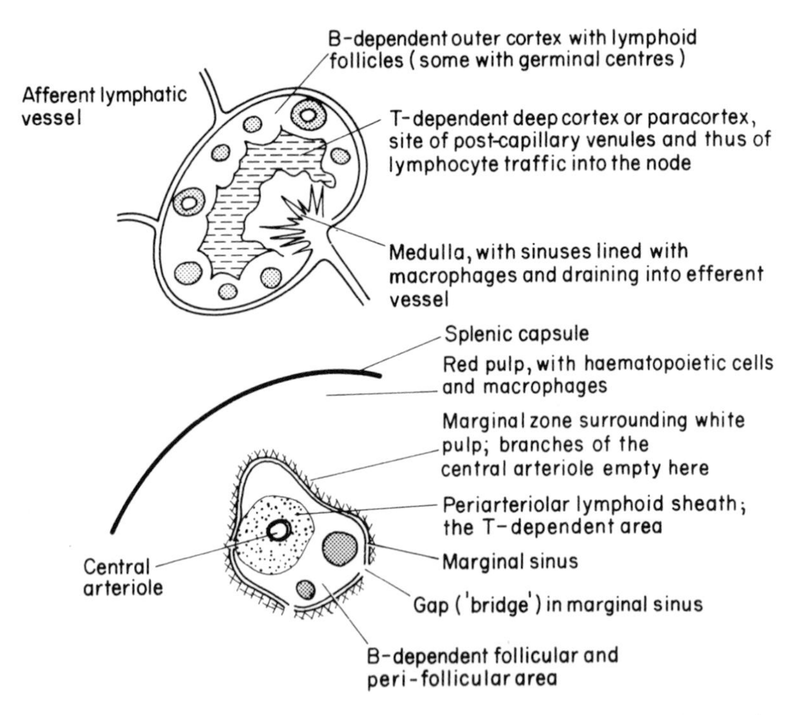

Fig. 4–4 Architecture of cross sections through a lymph node and part of a spleen to show the arrangement of T-dependent and B-dependent areas. Despite the concentration of small B-lymphocytes in the outer cortex of lymph nodes, their descendants, plasma cells, are located almost exclusively in the medulla.

of T-lymphocytes, while beyond this is the B-dependent area and a marginal zone which separates the areas of white pulp from the red pulp.

Within the B-dependent areas of both lymph nodes and spleen, the lymphoid follicles are characterized, during the development of antibody responses, by the localization of antigen and the presence of dividing lymphocytes. These dividing cells form the so-called germinal centres, and have been associated particularly with the generation and maintenance of immunological memory. The antigen is maintained on the finger-like processes of dendritic reticular cells which reach in among the clustered lymphocytes. The reticular cells obviously have the ability to take up antigen, but their relationship to conventional macrophages remains unclear.

The recirculation and tissue distribution of lymphocytes raises some interesting questions about cell–cell interactions in adult mammals or other vertebrates. The physiological basis for the change in life style from vagrant to temporary or permanent resident, and the molecular mechanisms by which T- and B-lymphocytes separate out in the lymphoid tissues, or recognize post-capillary venules, remain largely matters for conjecture, but the presence of antigens in these tissues is certainly an important factor in regulating the length of their stay.

4.6 Lymphoid tissue and the immune response

4.6.1 The fate of antigen in lymphoid tissues

When a particulate antigen such as sheep erythrocytes or bacteriophage T4 is injected into a mouse most of it will be taken up by phagocytic cells of the reticulo-endothelial system within a short period of time. These phagocytes are associated particularly with the spleen, lymph nodes, liver, lungs and with the mesenteries of the peritoneal cavity, and the exact distribution of antigen will depend on its route of administration. An intravenous injection of 8×10^8 particles of T4 is followed by removal of over 99.99 % of the antigen from the blood within 30 minutes, mostly by macrophages in the liver (Kupffer cells) and spleen. On the other hand, subcutaneous administration of such an antigen to a localized site results in its uptake by macrophages in the draining lymph nodes, although some antigen may also find its way to the liver and spleen, depending on the dose injected.

The mechanism by which vertebrate phagocytes recognize foreignness is not well understood. However a crucial step in the process of phagocytosis is adherence of an antigenic molecule to the phagocyte surface, and it seems likely that adherence and recognition are related events. It has been suggested that both electrostatic charge and the arrangement of sugar residues on the antigenic surface are important in binding by phagocytes. It is also clear that in mammalian macrophages, at least, recognition and adherence is enhanced in the presence of some classes of antibody which are able to bind to specific sites on the macrophage surface. Antibody–antigen complexes are thus easily attached and phagocytosed. The importance of antibody in contributing to antigen clearance is shown by the sequence of events which follow intravenous injection of a soluble antigen, such as a non-aggregated protein. Removal from the blood is relatively slow for 6 or 7 days, then the rate of clearance shows a sharp increase, coincident with the secretion by lymphocytes of the first specific antibody. This second phase is known as the period of immune clearance.

Once ingested, most antigen is rapidly broken down by intracellular enzymes, but since degradation follows either a biphasic or an exponential pattern small amounts often persist for very long periods of time. By the use of radio-isotopically-labelled antigens in rodents it has been estimated that some of the injected material survives for a year or more. Some of this long-lived antigen is found on the surface of the dendritic reticular cells of lymphoid follicles, and may also be associated with macrophage membranes. Its presence is important in the long-term regulation of antibody production, and in the generation and maintenance of immunological memory.

Antibody also influences the localization of antigen in lymphoid follicles. In a true primary response, antigen is associated only with macrophages until the first antibody has been produced. On the other hand, administration of specific antibody (prepared in another animal) together with the antigen results in the antigen's rapid appearance on dendritic reticular cells. Similar rapid localization in the follicles is seen if antigen is injected into a previously immunized animal which already has at least some antibody in its blood stream.

4.6.2 Lymphocyte localization

It has been pointed out that lymphocytes are essentially a recirculating population, migrating from blood to spleen and back, or from blood to lymph via the post-capillary venules and the tissues of the lymph nodes. This behavioural pattern greatly increases the likelihood of the 'correct' lymphocytes encountering localized antigen, and ensures the body-wide distribution of memory cells. It is now clear, from experiments using lymphocytes labelled with radio-isotopes, that after the arrival of an antigen, physiological changes take place in lymphoid tissues which increase their lymphocyte content. Following injection of labelled syngeneic lymphocytes, comparisons between draining and non-draining lymph nodes show more radio-activity in the former, and therefore more cells. (*Syngeneic* cells are obtained from other mice of the same inbred strain. They are thus genetically identical with recipients into which they are transferred, and not antigenic. Contrast *allogeneic* cells which are obtained from genetically dissimilar members of the same species, and *xenogeneic* cells from a different species. Hence also *allograft* and *xenograft*.)

This observation applies equally to the administration of an antigen such as sheep erythrocytes and to a graft of foreign tissue such as skin, although the time scale of events is somewhat different. The degree of localization of labelled lymphocytes is dependent upon the dose of antigen and reflects the transient accumulation of normal host cells at the site of antigen localization, since it can be shown that the injected radio-labelled cells enter the recirculating pool and act as a marker for the distribution and behaviour of host lymphocytes.

The first explanation given for this phenomenon was that lymphocytes entering the draining lymph node were 'trapped' there, and thus accumulated within the tissue of the node. It was suggested that, among all those lymphocytes whose progress was thus arrested by this 'road block' effect, some would be specific for the antigen and these could then more easily be brought into the response by reaction with macrophage-borne antigen. However, some recent experiments have thrown doubt on this explanation, by showing firstly that exit of lymphocytes from an antigenically stimulated lymph node is not markedly reduced, except for a very brief period shortly after the localization of antigen, and, secondly that the blood flow to draining lymphoid organs is temporarily increased. Since the number of lymphocytes entering the tissues of a lymph node is proportional to the number flowing through in the blood stream, it now seems likely that lymphocyte accumulation after antigen injection is largely explained in terms of local changes in blood flow. It is not known how these variations are induced, although there is evidence that macrophages may have a role in their initiation.

5 Cellular Events in Antibody Production

The key event in the induction of antibody synthesis, as in other categories of immune response, is the interaction of antigen with lymphocyte surface receptors. B-lymphocyte receptors were shown in Chapter 4 to be immunoglobulins which vary in class according to the stage of maturation of the cell, but which are identical, in terms of antigen specificity, to the antibodies which that cell will produce once stimulated. According to the theory of clonal selection, antigen binds to and selects only those B-cells bearing complementary receptors. The selected lymphocytes then multiply up into clones of memory cells and antibody-secreting plasma cells. In this way the specificity of the response is assured.

T-lymphocytes are likewise equipped with receptors, and since some of these have been shown to have idiotypic identity with both B-cell receptors and circulating antibodies, it may be assumed that the T-cell receptor includes immunoglobulin V-region sequences. However, it has proved more difficult to demonstrate the T-cell receptor than to investigate its B-cell counterpart, and the precise nature of the receptor molecule remains in doubt. Observations suggesting that T-lymphocytes possess surface immunoglobulin of T-cell origin have always been controversial, and present evidence is best interpreted as showing that the receptor is part immunoglobulin V-region, part product of the major histocompatibility complex (MHC, see Chapter 6). It comprises, as it were, the business end of an antibody (most probably V_H) coupled to a non-immunoglobulin backbone.

The non-immunoglobulin portion of the T-cell receptor appears to play an important role in many antibody responses. Observations suggesting that related molecules are released from stimulated T-cells and participate in the activation of B-cells (thus mediating T-cell 'help') are discussed in section 5.4. One mechanism involves the binding of the T-cell factor to the B-lymphocyte membrane together with antigen, and implies that stimulation of B-cells may be a two step process involving surface receptors for molecules other than antigen.

5.1 Lymphocyte proliferation

Among the earliest changes shown by B-lymphocytes following antigenic stimulation are enlargement, RNA and DNA synthesis, and cell division. Cell division in particular has a most important role to play in the development of humoral immunity, firstly because it allows a small number of precursor cells to provide an adequate response, and secondly, because memory cells as well as antibody-forming cells result from the divisions taking place within each stimulated clone.

Proliferation of lymphocytes may be detected by the technique of injecting radio-isotopically-labelled nucleotides which are incorporated into the DNA of dividing cells. If mice immunized by intravenous injection of sheep erythrocytes are treated in this way, and the amount of radioactivity in their spleens is measured, it is found that increased cell division follows directly after peak lymphocyte accumulation (see Chapter 4), and reaches a peak itself 48–72 hours after immunization Fig. 5–1). By using transfused lymphocytes carrying distinctive chromosomes (which allows dividing cells to be identified as to their origin, if observed at metaphase), it can also be shown that T-

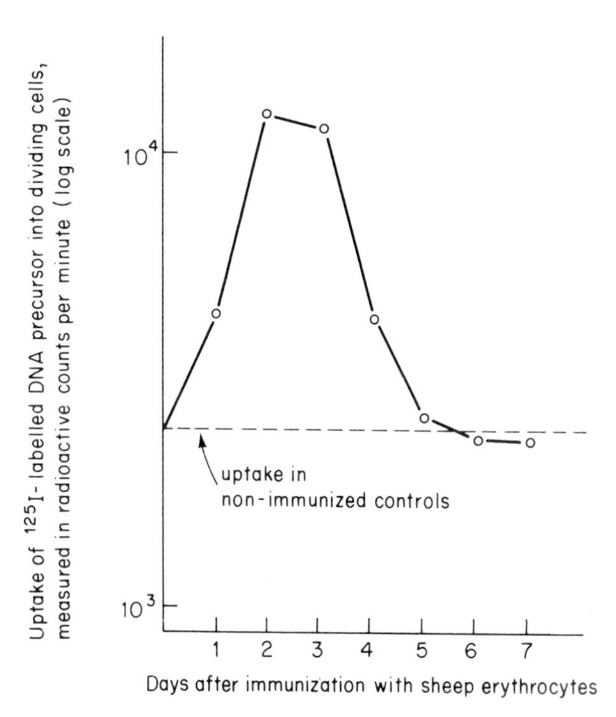

Fig. 5–1 Proliferative response of splenic lymphocytes following immunization of mice with sheep erythrocytes.

lymphocytes divide early in the response while peak proliferation of B-cells follows later.

The proliferative phase of an antibody response precedes antibody production itself, but its effect on antibody production can be clearly seen if antibody-forming cells are enumerated at intervals after immunization. The haemolytic plaque assay, for instance, has been widely used in research to measure responses to foreign erythrocytes (Fig. 5–2) and gives a direct indication of the numbers of antibody-secreting plasma cells when the numbers of plaque-forming cells (PFC) are counted. If the spleens of mice immunized intravenously with sheep erythrocytes are examined in this way, raised levels of PFC are detected within 48 hours of immunization, and after 4 days, as many as 2×10^5 PFC per spleen are observed. Since anti-mitotic drugs greatly suppress PFC formation, it can be seen that the response develops mainly by cell

(a) A mouse is immunized intravenously with
a suspension of sheep erythrocytes

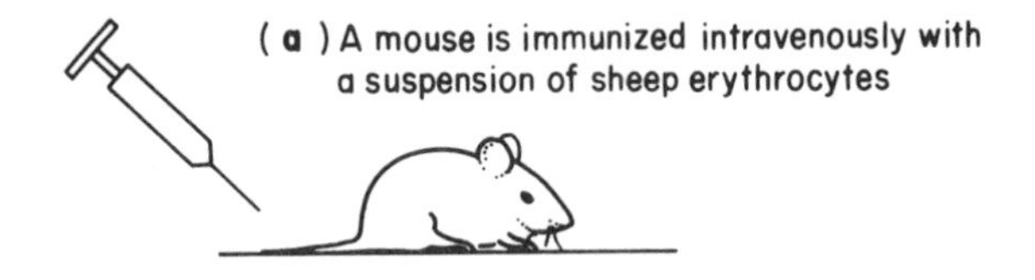

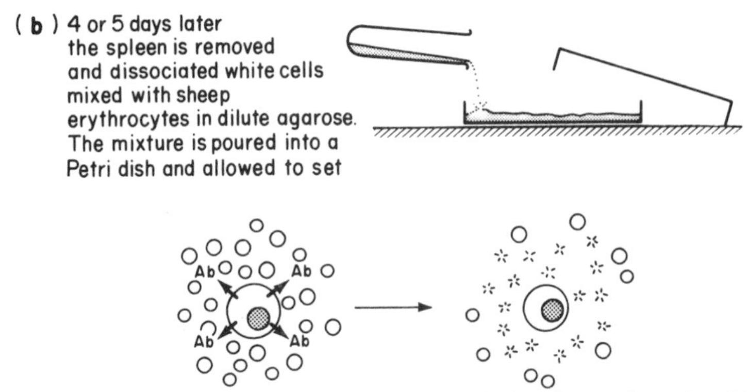

Fig. 5–2 The haemolytic plaque assay is a convenient way of measuring numbers of specific antibody-forming cells in the response to erythrocyte antigens, or to haptens which can be coupled to erythrocyte surfaces. The technique as shown measures IgM-forming cells, but it can be adapted to detect IgG-secreting cells also. The assay may also be performed on microscope slides, in which case a liquid medium can be used.

division from a small number of precursor cells (it should be made clear that these precursor cells are not the same as the 100 or so 'background' PFC usually observed in laboratory mice, since plasma cells are usually regarded as 'end cells').

Proliferation is thus an important characteristic of responding lymphocytes, not only in antibody responses but in graft rejection and other aspects of cell-mediated immunity as well. In tissue culture, both B- and T-lymphocytes similarly respond to antigens by dividing, and this property has become the basis of the tests for cellular compatibility which are standard procedure before grafting in human patients.

The termination of the proliferative phase in the intact animal has been taken by many to indicate the activity of regulatory or suppressor cells whose function is to control the scope of each immune response. Their activities are discussed at a later stage in this chapter.

5.2 Antibody synthesis

Inspection of an unstimulated B-lymphocyte reveals it to be an unlikely candidate for a major producer of extracellular proteins. Virgin B-lymphocytes are small cells, with rather sparse cytoplasm, and little in the way of endoplasmic reticulum, Golgi apparatus, or the other paraphernalia of protein synthesis. It therefore follows that major intracellular re-organization takes place from the moment that the newly stimulated B-cell first starts to enlarge into the characteristic intermediate stage, the lymphoblast (Fig. 5–3). Thus, along with cell division, there is a great increase in the amount of intracellular membrane, the Golgi apparatus becomes prominent, and histochemical techniques reveal the synthesis of large amounts of RNA.

The typical antibody-producing end cell, the plasma cell, has, in consequence, well developed rough endoplasmic reticulum where antibody H and L chains are separately manufactured (Fig. 5–3). Free L chains, but not free H chains, are found in the cisternae of the endoplasmic reticulum, since the first step in the assembly of a complete antibody molecule is the addition of one L chain to one H chain at the H chain polyribosome. Subsequent joining of H–L dimers results in the formation of whole molecules which, following the addition of carbohydrate side chains, pass via the Golgi apparatus to the plasma membrane. Here they are released into the tissue fluids and so to the blood. It should be noted that B-cell membrane (receptor) immunoglobulin is produced in the same manner and at a rate which maintains about 10^4 receptor molecules per cell. However, it seems likely that receptor antibodies derive from a special messenger RNA which codes for an additional peptide sequence at the COOH-terminal end of the H chain. This extra sequence has the postulated function of ensuring the

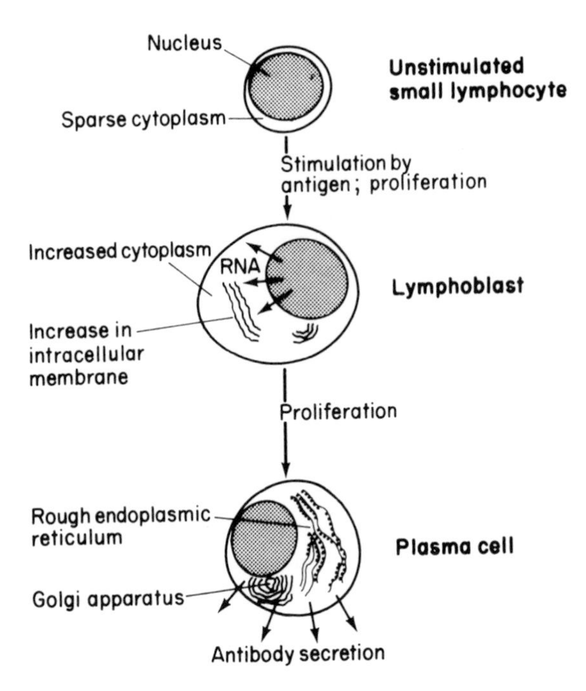

Fig. 5–3 Stages in the generation of an antibody-forming plasma cell from a B-lymphocyte precursor.

stability of receptor molecules within the membrane. The balance between production of secretory and receptor antibody in B-cells remains an interesting area for investigation not just for the immunologist, but for cell biologists generally.

Another interesting aspect of antibody production in higher vertebrates is the diversity of antibody classes, and the sequential manufacture of the two major types, IgM and IgG, in most antibody responses (the main exception being the production of IgM only in response to certain polysaccharide antigens). IgM is generally the first antibody to appear (Fig. 5–4), although analysis of antibody-forming cells rather than serum antibodies now suggests that IgG is manufactured rather earlier in the response than was once thought. It has been a matter for debate whether IgM and IgG molecules of identical specificity for antigen are produced sequentially by single clones of B-lymphocytes. This view is generally favoured, but what causes the switch in antibody production is unknown. The evidence for the secretion of both IgM and IgG by a single plasma cell, either simultaneously or sequentially, is slight.

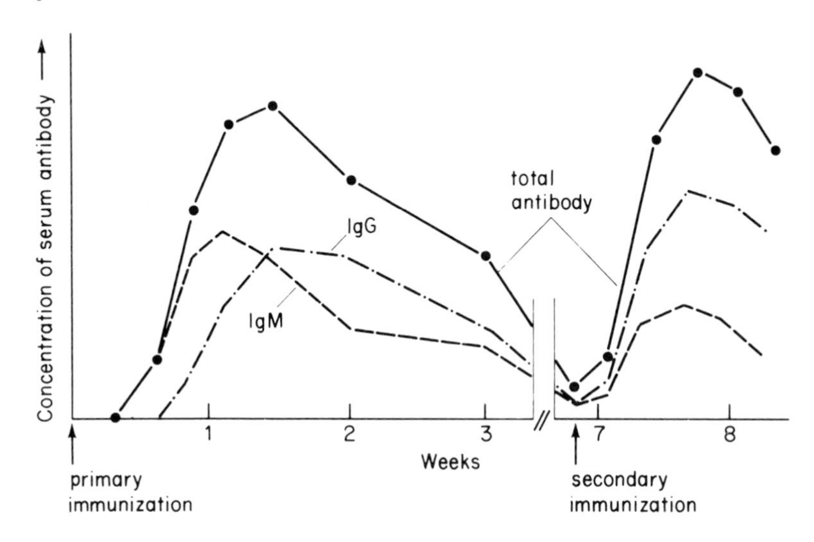

Fig. 5–4 Hypothetical antibody response to illustrate the production of IgM (————) and IgG (—·—·—) antibodies in primary and secondary responses. Note the shorter lag period and the faster rise in antibody titre which is characteristic of secondary responses. With some antigens, primary responses develop more slowly than shown here, while with others, prolonged IgG synthesis after a single immunizing injection may give rise to high antibody titres several weeks after immunization.

5.3 Cell interactions in antibody production

It is now well established for antibody responses to most antigens that the precursor B-lymphocyte is but one member of a team of interacting cells, and that stimulation of B-cells by antigen and their subsequent behaviour come under the influence of other cell types. Chief among these are, firstly, macrophages which process and present antigen to lymphocytes, and secondly, T-lymphocytes, in the roles of both helper and suppressor cell. These two categories of T-cell can now be clearly distinguished by the presence on their cell membranes of different subsets of the Lyt differentiation antigens: Lyt $1^+2^-3^-$ for helpers; Lyt 2^+3^+ (with perhaps small amounts of Lyt 1) for suppressors.

The classic experiments of J. F. A. P. Miller and his colleagues throughout the 1960s led to the identification of T- and B-cells as distinct classes of lymphocyte, and also indicated the essential part played by helper T-cells in many antibody responses. It was shown that mice thymectomized at birth were not only unable to reject skin grafts, but also gave greatly reduced antibody responses to commonly used antigens such as sheep erythrocytes or heterologous serum proteins (thymectomy had to be at birth since certain classes of T-lymphocyte are long-lived cells, and the effects of adult thymectomy are not noticed for long periods of time). If, on the other hand, thymectomized animals were given injections of syngeneic thymus or thoracic duct lymphocytes in adult life, their ability to make antibodies was restored, although it was found that the donor T-cells were not actually responsible for antibody synthesis. This observation has been widely confirmed in thymectomized and irradiated mice, where both T- and B-lymphocytes must be given to reconstitute the recipients, and also in tissue culture, where the accessory role of both macrophages and T-cells is clearly demonstrated.

The manner in which T-lymphocytes help in the stimulation of precursor B-cells remains uncertain, despite the great deal of attention which has been focused on this problem in the last ten years or so. But some useful pointers have emerged, the first among them resulting from the use of thymectomized, irradiated and reconstituted mice which were immunized with haptens coupled to protein carriers. It was found that secondary anti-hapten responses in recipient mice only resulted if the transferred lymphocytes contained T-cells primed against the carrier; that is, when donor T- and B-cells were taken from mice previously immunized respectively with carrier alone and with hapten coupled to an unrelated carrier (Fig. 5–5). Thus there is an important element of specificity about T-lymphocyte help but, for any given antigenic determinant, it is directed against other parts of the whole antigenic molecule; against carrier determinants rather than the hapten. It was first suggested that T-lymphocytes functioned by focusing antigen directly on to the B-cell surface, but evidence that T-lymphocytes can help B-lymphocytes in culture when separated from them by a cell-impermeable membrane suggests that some T-cell-derived factor is involved rather than cell–cell contact. This, of course, implies that B-cells need some signal in addition to the simple presence of antigen before they can be 'switched on'.

5.4 Cellular mechanisms in T-cell–B-cell cooperation

What is the nature of the T-lymphocyte helper factor, and its influence on B-lymphocyte stimulation? It would be agreeable to be able to set down a single well-proven model, but at present that is not possible. Rather there is evidence for a number of plausible, but not absolutely convincing, theories and, provided that the truth does not lie somewhere between them all, it seems correct to conclude that B-cells may be activated by more than one mechanism.

Three major categories of factor have been isolated from helper T-

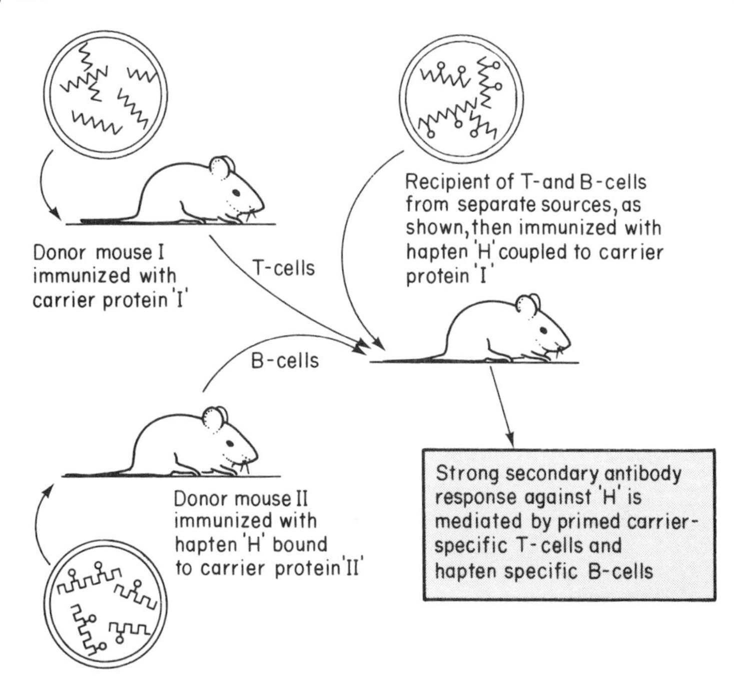

Fig. 5–5 Cell transfer experiment illustrating the 'carrier effect', and demonstrating the role of T-lymphocytes in responding to carrier determinants. Control groups in the experiment show that only weak (primary) responses result in the recipient if the donor T-cells have not 'seen' the carrier 'I' molecule before, or the B-cells hapten 'H'.

cells, two of them specific for antigen, and one non-specific. The latter shows no antigen-binding ability and contributes to the stimulation of B-cells regardless of their own antigen specificity. There is no incongruity about this suggestion, since the specificity of the response is preserved by the requirements for T-cell activation in the first place, and is undoubtedly aided in the intact animal by the close association of responding T- and B-cells. Originally, evidence for non-specific helper factor came from experiments in which T-lymphocytes were first cultured with foreign (allogeneic) cells and the cell-free supernates then added to B-lymphocytes in the presence of antigen. 'Allogeneic effect factor' (AEF) in the culture supernates proved to be able to substitute for T-cells and help B-cells to make antibody against quite unrelated antigens (Fig. 5–6). AEF has been partially characterized in mice, and has been identified as a product of the I region of the MHC, a part of the

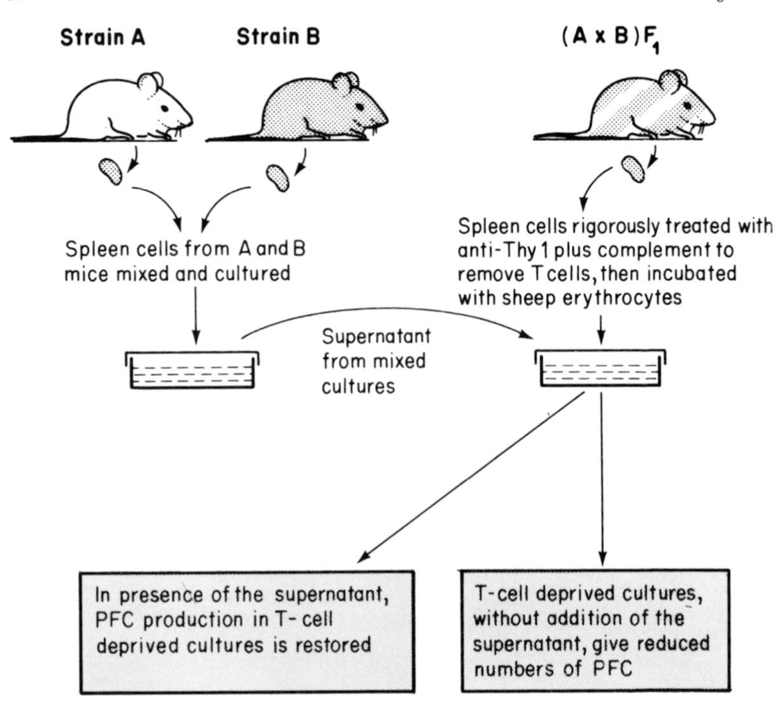

Fig. 5–6 'Allogeneic effect factor' is produced by T-cells when allogeneic lymphocytes (from different strains of mice) are mixed. This factor is able to substitute for T-cell help in antibody responses, and promotes the production of antibody-forming cells from antigen-stimulated B-lymphocytes. Note that lymphocyte surface antigens which stimulate factor formation in the first culture are quite unrelated to the antigenic determinants on sheep erythrocytes, so this effect is non-specific.

genome which is intimately concerned with the control of both cell surface and immunologically active molecules (see Chapter 6).

The evidence for two categories of antigen-specific factor depends on slightly conflicting observations from mouse experiments in which different antigens and procedures were used. Although both types of factor bind antigen, one is reported to be an immunoglobulin, while the other is a non-immunoglobulin molecule consisting, at least in part, of a product of the MHC I-region. It is impossible to say at present why, in each experiment, the alternative factor was not produced, or was overlooked.

The immunoglobulin-like factor receives best support from the work of Feldmann in the early 1970s, as a result of experiments in which primed T-cells and antigen, in one chamber, were cultured next to B-cells, macrophages and antigen in an adjacent chamber. The two chambers were separated by a cell impermeable membrane which allowed the free passage of molecules in solution. Only when both chambers contained their proper complement of cells plus antigen were the B-cells stimulated to make antibody. The procedure is shown in Fig. 5–7, which also shows the interpretation placed on these results. The T-cell helper factor, identified as an immunoglobulin ('IgT'), is believed to become absorbed onto macrophage membranes where it binds antigen in a 'critical matrix' at sufficient concentration to stimulate B-cells. A weakness of this model lies in the fact that it has been clearly shown that macrophages, after first encounter with antigen, process it themselves and present it in such a way as to stimulate T-lymphocytes.

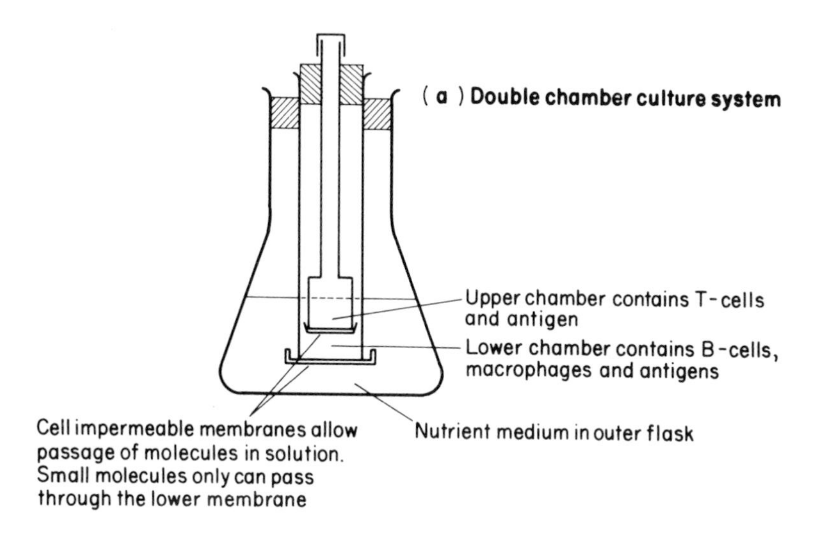

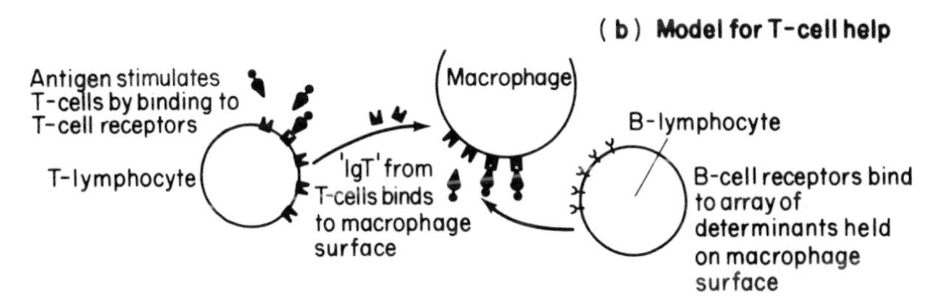

Fig. 5–7 The 'IgT' model of T-lymphocyte help (apparatus redrawn after Feldmann and Basten (1972). *J. exp. Med.*, **136**, 49).

Furthermore, antibodies are made against the degradation products of many antigens. If macrophage surface-bound antigen is available anyway, it is difficult to see why 'IgT' is needed.

The second model of antigen-specific help derives from experiments reported by Munro and Taussig in 1974, in which a factor, produced in culture by antigen-stimulated T-cells, was able to substitute for T-cells when injected with antigen into irradiated, B-cell-repopulated recipient mice. This factor failed to react with anti-mouse Ig antibodies, but combined with antibodies against MHC I region products. It therefore bears considerable resemblance to the postulated T-lymphocyte receptor described earlier in this chapter. The factor was also shown to be absorbed out of culture supernates by incubation with B-cells. There is thus a B-cell acceptor for this helper substance (Fig. 5–8), and the acceptor has also been identified as an MHC I region product. Presumably, if similar acceptors existed on macrophage membranes, as has been proposed by some workers, this second factor could also bind antigen at the macrophage surface and so focus it for presentation to B-cells in a manner similar to that described for IgT.

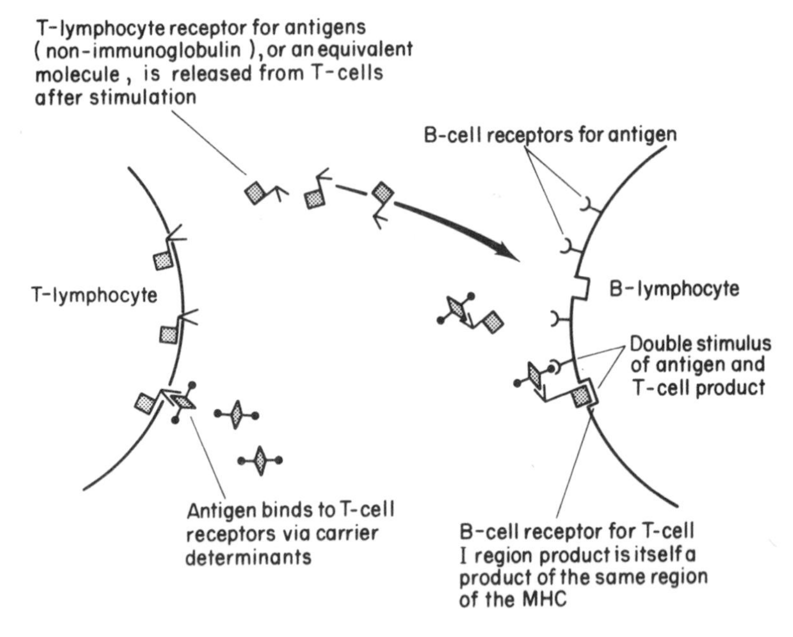

Fig. 5–8 Co-operation model involving products of the MHC (after Munro and Taussig (1975) *Nature*, **256**, 103). The factor could locate on other cell surfaces, e.g. macrophages, provided receptors exist.

Both these models are, in a sense, victims of the difficulties experienced in culture work of this sort and of the problems in developing reliable assays for the exact nature and function of soluble factors. Both the experiments and their interpretation are being updated continually in the scientific literature. Munro has described such experiments as 'temperamental' and they need to be interpreted with caution, particularly with regard to their reflection of events in the intact animal. Nevertheless, the second of these antigen-specific models has two particular merits: the factor has been shown to work *in vivo*, and the requirement for I region products links well with other experiments which associate genetically-determined immune capability with genes in the I region (immune-response, or Ir, genes). Thus the differences, observed with some antigens, between low and high responder strains of mouse or guinea pig may be explained on the basis of inherited deficiencies in T-cell receptors or B-cell acceptors. In this general area it is now important to establish what link exists between the Ir genes inferred from genetical experiments and the functional I region products such as those described above.

The difficulties with the models of B-cell stimulation do not end with the discrepancies between the various factors, since three different mechanisms of B-cell stimulation are also implied. The IgT model depends on a single signal, provided by antigen in sufficient concentration, and this view is supported by the fact that antigens with identical repeating determinants are much less dependent on T-cell help than are antigens which show little or no epitope duplication. On the other hand, both the remaining models require a 'second signal'. This additional signal is independent of antigen in the case of AEF, but bound to it in the case of the I region factor. We also know that polymeric antigens (particularly polysaccharides) are capable of stimulating B-cells directly without T-cell help, usually giving rise to a response which consists of IgM alone. These observations indicate another T-cell function, control of IgG synthesis, but they also remind us again that B-cells can in fact be stimulated under a variety of different conditions, and that no single model can claim to portray the whole story.

5.5 Regulation of antibody production

Three important factors combine to regulate the production of antibody during the course of an immune response. They are (*i*) the activities of T-lymphocytes, (*ii*) the long term persistence of antigen, and (*iii*) serum antibody levels.

In addition to helper T-cells, whose role in initiation of antibody synthesis and in regulating antibody class has already been discussed, there are also subpopulations of T-lymphocytes which have an inhibitory function. These cells are identified not only by their functional characteristics but by morphological markers such as the presence of Lyt 2, 3 determinants on the cell surface. Their effect in the whole animal is most easily seen with responses to antigens such as bacterial polysaccharides which do not need T-cell help to induce antibody formation (the so-called T-independent antigens). These responses may be *increased* in size if steps are first taken to deplete the experimental animal of all T-lymphocytes, due to the fact that the active suppressor subpopulation is also removed.

Experiments with cultured cells have revealed the existence of soluble factors, derived from suppressor T-cells, which are able to switch off the proliferative responses of other lymphocytes. Factors such as these could obviously be responsible for the termination of cell division in the intact animal (see section 5.1 and Fig. 5–1), thus limiting the amount of antibody produced and controlling overstimulation by antigen. Suppressor activity can be either antigen specific or lacking in specificity, depending on the circumstances of immunization. In the latter instance, products of stimulated suppressor cells are potentially capable of inhibiting responses to unrelated antigens, and the fact that general immunosuppression throughout the body does not normally occur is probably due to the localized production of suppressor factors and a restriction upon the area of their activity. In contrast, T-cells which mediate specific suppression are also responsible for some manifestations of immunological tolerance, in which an animal is temporarily or even permanently deprived of the ability to respond to a particular antigen (see section 6.3).

The roles of persisting antigen and circulating antibody in controlling antibody production are closely linked, and the long term progress of an antibody response is dependent upon the balance between these two factors. It has been shown, for instance, that if antibody levels in an immunized rabbit are substantially reduced by blood transfusion, as when antibody-rich blood is replaced by blood from an unimmunized donor, then a burst of new antibody synthesis follows so as to restore the antibody titre to its 'correct' level. On the other hand, if the transfused blood contains an equal amount of antibody to that removed, then little or no fresh synthesis results. It is therefore apparent that overall antibody output is determined by the total level of serum antibody, and the most likely explanation of the mechanism is that there exists an equilibrium in the immunized animal between residual antigen (possibly on macrophage surfaces), lymphocyte receptors for antigen, and circulating antibody. In the steady state, antibody combines with the antigen, thus restricting lymphocyte access, but if the antibody level drops, the antigen is uncovered and available lymphocytes are stimulated afresh. This hypothesis has been elegantly supported by experiments in which lymph nodes were removed from rabbits several months after immunization and their constituent cells cultured without addition of further antigen. Spontaneous bursts of antibody synthesis were seen in the cultures, but these were suppressed if small amounts of specific antibody were added. It was argued that washing of the lymph node cells prior to culture removed native antibody and thus opened the way for residual antigen to restimulate available lymphocytes. It is known that some antigens persist for very long periods of time in an active form and this may provide an explanation for the prolonged protection given by some inoculations.

5.6 Immunological memory

A characteristic feature of specific immune responses, whether cellular or humoral, which distinguishes them from non-specific immunity, is the development of immunological memory. This property results in secondary antibody responses having a shorter lag period before the first appearance of antibody and a much sharper rise in the numbers of antibody-forming cells and in the serum titre. Peak antibody titres are often greater than for a primary response, but this is not always the case, and in some instances may be due as much to increased antibody affinity as to increased molecular concentration in the blood. With the exception of those responses where IgG is never produced, and in contrast to primary responses, IgG is usually the predominant antibody in secondary responses with peak levels of IgG-forming cells exceeding peak IgM production (Fig. 5–4).

The rate of development of immunological memory after primary immunization varies according to the antigen used. With particulate or cellular antigens such as heterologous erythrocytes, memory cells are rapidly produced and can be detected in the circulation of the mouse 4–5 days after intraperitoneal immunization. With protein antigens, memory takes longer to become established, and its development has been shown to depend on the continued presence of antigen. In a similar manner, the duration of immunological memory varies from antigen to antigen, a fact which is reflected in the different intervals at which we need to receive booster injections of the common inoculations. Why a single dose of one antigen should confer life-long immunity, while others give only temporary protection remains something of a mystery. However, it is unlikely that lymphocytes of different specificities vary in their life span, and more probable that it has to do with the rate at which different antigens are eliminated from the body. Those antigens which survive the longest should produce the most persistent memory, since

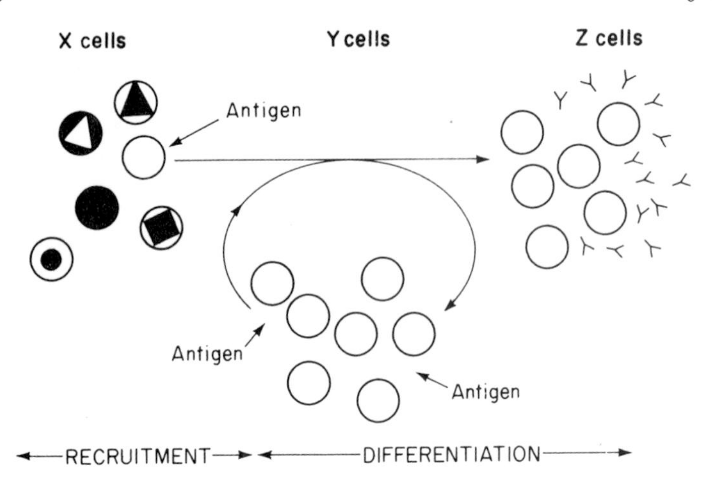

Fig. 5-9 The X–Y–Z scheme of B-lymphocyte differentiation through to antibody-producing plasma cells. Memory (Y) cells are shown below the main pathway. Antigen is involved both in the maintenance of the memory cell pool and in the recruitment of memory cells back into the main plasma cell pathway.

the low-level antigenic stimulation which results will keep the memory population 'topped up' for long periods of time.

Immunological memory is characteristic of both T- and B-lymphocytes, including those T-lymphocytes which cooperate in humoral responses. The basis of B-cell memory is to be found in three major differences which distinguish the primed from the unprimed animal, the first of these being simply that priming results in the presence of many more responsive cells as a consequence of lymphocyte proliferation. As has been mentioned before, each lymphocyte clone consists not only of antibody-forming cells but also of memory cells generated during clonal expansion, and particularly after low doses of antigen the balance will be in favour of more memory cells and less antibody producers. Conversely, if large priming doses are used, memory is often less well developed, probably because a proportion of B-memory cells will mature to antibody-forming cells during the primary response itself, stimulated by the high concentration of antigen.

In addition to the increased numbers of memory cells, priming also favours selection of lymphocytes bearing receptors of highest affinity for the antigen used. This point, together with the fact that memory cells seem to have a greater density of receptors than their unprimed counterparts, enables primed lymphocytes to 'see' antigen more rapidly and efficiently. Thus the characteristic advantages of secondary responses are obtained.

Finally, the presence of small amounts of pre-existing antibody in primed animals also contributes to the rapid onset of secondary humoral responses due to the fact that antigen is localized more quickly in the lymphoid tissues, and particularly in lymphoid follicles, in the presence of specific antibody.

What then is the relationship of B-memory cells to the unstimulated B-lymphocyte on the one hand, and to the antibody-producing plasma cell on the other? A simple view is that they form three stages of a linear progression, X, Y and Z, the Y cell representing the memory cell. However, since memory cells are small lymphocytes, similar in appearance to unstimulated X cells, they must at some point diverge from the line of large proliferating blastoid cells which progress directly to antibody formation and secretion. It is therefore more satisfactory to regard memory cells as a side pathway, into which many members of each clone are diverted during proliferation and differentiation (Fig. 5–9). What causes particular cells to enter this alternative pathway and remain there until restimulated by antigen is unknown.

6 Cell-mediated Immunity, Tolerance and Allergies

6.1 Grafts and tumours

Rejection of transplanted tissue is now known to be a feature of both invertebrate and vertebrate immune systems, and is one of the reasons for suspecting that lymphocytes have a history which goes back beyond the chordates (see Chapter 2). In man and other mammals, clinical experience has shown that the efficiency of the rejection response is a major barrier to transplant surgery, frustrating attempts to exchange new parts for old, and making careful tissue matching and the use of immunosuppressive drugs absolutely essential.

Among the mammals, however, there are some exceptions to the rule that tissue grafts are rejected and these provide useful pointers to the mechanisms which contribute to rejection. Firstly, grafts of self tissue, as often happens in plastic surgery or treatment for burns, or grafts from a genetically identical donor generally succeed. Thus transplants between members of a single inbred strain of mice are accepted. Similarly in man, kidneys grafted from one identical twin to another were among the first successful renal transplants, and (since not many of us have identical twins) close relatives are often preferred as tissue donors due to their strong genetic resemblance to the patient.

Secondly, dead or non-vascularized tissue can frequently be transplanted without fear of immune rejection; corneal transplants are a good example of such an operation and tissue-matching of donor and recipient is not necessary. Then there are various places in the body, known as immunologically privileged sites, where grafts of living foreign tissue will succeed, despite obvious antigenicity. One of the first of these to be exploited experimentally was the hamster cheek pouch. In general these sites are characterized by a lack of lymphatic drainage, so that there is no channel by which antigenic material from the graft can make its way to an adjacent lymph node.

These observations give certain clues to the sequence of events in graft rejection. Due to genetic differences between donor and host, a tissue allograft (that is, from a non-identical member of the same species; see p. 41) will carry cell surface molecules which are antigenic to the host and some of these, normally products of the MHC, are particularly good at provoking lymphocytes into a rejection response. Taking a skin graft as an example, there is usually a period lasting two or three days during which blood supply to the transplant and lymphatic drainage from its immediate environment are established. Before long however, cellular debris from the graft is able to pass in the lymph to the draining lymph node where a familiar sequence of events occurs – lymphocyte 'trapping' (see section 4.5) and then proliferation of specifically-responding cells. Since graft rejection is primarily an expression of cell-mediated immunity, particularly with solid transplants such as skin, the stimulation of T-lymphocytes is the crucial event. Although anti-graft antibodies may form, they normally appear later in the response, and contribute most to the rejection of transplants with a well developed innate blood supply, for example kidney. With grafts such as skin, the cellular basis of the response has been clearly shown in mice by the fact that transfused T-cells can confer immunity against a graft on an unimmunized recipient, but that injections of serum from the same source have little effect (Fig. 6–1).

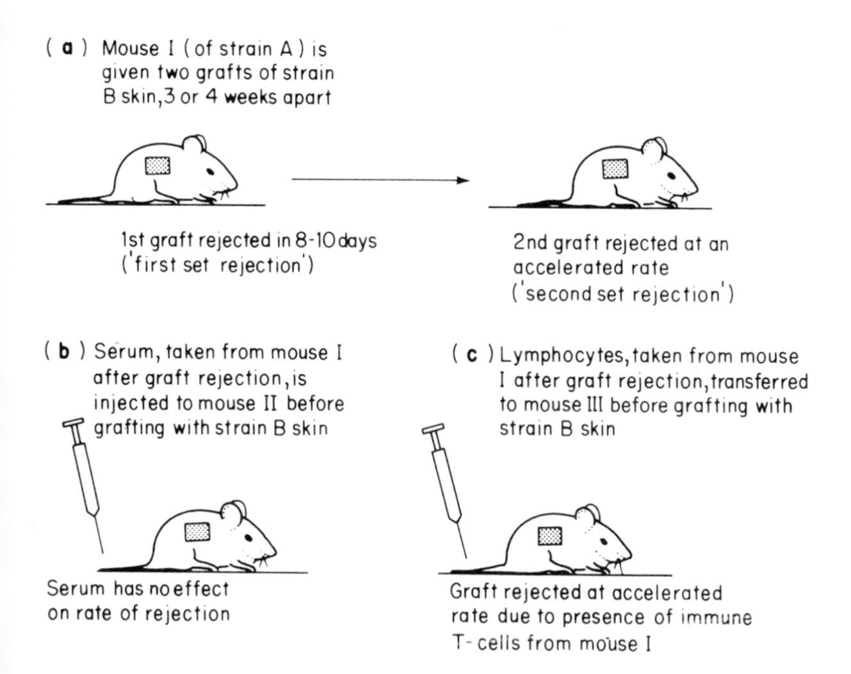

Fig. 6–1 Cellular basis of skin graft rejection in mice of strain A grafted with strain B skin. Lymphocyte involvement is shown by the presence of immunological memory in mouse I after the first graft. Only transferred cells from mouse I are able to confer immunity on unimmunised mice (II and III). Transfer of serum has little or no effect.

In a similar manner to that described for B-lymphocytes, stimulation of T-cells by graft antigens results in clonal expansion and the appearance of both memory cells and effector cells. These committed lymphocytes re-enter the circulation, and, in the latter case, begin to make their appearance at the site of the graft itself. Infiltration of the graft by mononuclear cells, mainly T-lymphocytes and macrophages, is the first indication that the rejection process has begun. There is little evidence at this stage of either granulocytes or plasma cells. T-cells are localized presumably as a result of interaction between graft antigens and T-cell receptors, and the response then develops in one of two ways. In the first case, T-lymphocytes themselves mature to become functional cytotoxic cells, with binding of lymphocytes to target cell antigens resulting very shortly in the death of the graft. The generation of cytotoxic T-cells can be reproduced in culture, the normal starting point being the 'one way' mixed lymphocyte reaction (MLR) in which two populations of genetically distinct lymphocytes are mixed (Fig. 6–2). While the responder population proliferates, giving rise to cytotoxic cells, the target population is inhibited from giving its own reciprocal response by prior treatment with a drug such as mitomycin C. Close examination of the MLR shows that the generation of cytotoxic cells, whose presence is detected in a subsequent assay (Fig. 6–2), depends on the presence and activity of a population of helper T-cells. In this respect there is a parallel between the induction of cell-mediated immunity and the antibody response to T-dependent antigens given by B-cells.

Once committed, T-lymphocytes are also able to initiate graft rejection by a second mechanism involving macrophages which are stimulated through the activity of soluble T-cell factors, often collectively referred to as *lymphokines*. Important among these are macrophage migration inhibition factor, and macrophage arming factors which include an antigen specific factor. Macrophages exposed to these factors are able to inhibit cell division in the transplant, and to kill grafted cells. The first of these responses is particularly important if the transplant consists of rapidly dividing tissue, such as a tumour (see below).

It has been mentioned that in some circumstances anti-graft antibodies are able to make a contribution to graft rejection. They may bring about the death of grafted tissue by the direct involvement of complement (see section 3.5), or by the activation of certain cells which develop cytotoxic function in the presence of antibody or antibody-antigen complexes. These cells include both macrophages and polymorphs, together with a family of cells called killer (K) cells which have certain similarities to B-cells, but whose relationship to the lymphocyte line is still uncertain. It should also be said that antibody can have the opposite effect, prolonging the survival of transplanted tissue

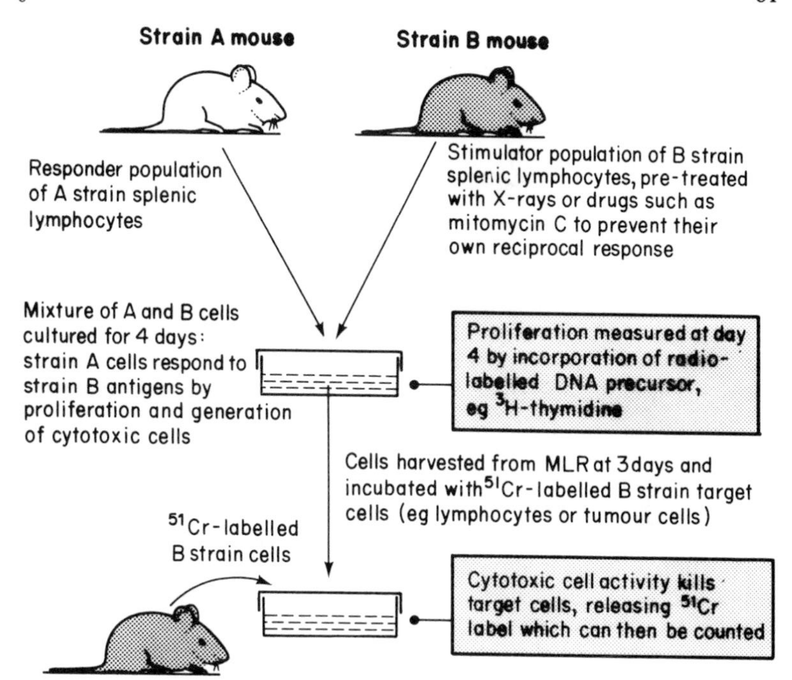

Fig. 6–2 Generation of cytotoxic T-cells during a mixed lymphocyte reaction. The degree of stimulation in the MLR is measured by the uptake of radioactive DNA precursors. The presence of cytotoxic cells is detected in a second assay during which cells harvested from the MLR are incubated with new targets in the form of ^{51}Cr-labelled B strain cells. The Cr label is released into the supernate when the target cells are killed, and the level of cytoxic cell activity can therefore be estimated.

and tumours. Such enhancing antibody may function by concealing antigenic determinants from the receptors on T-lymphocytes, either at the induction or at the effector (cytolytic) stage of the response. Obviously the antibody must not bind in such a way as to stimulate complement-dependent or K-cell cytolysis, and the story is complicated by the fact that enhancing factors, when isolated, generally prove to be antibody–antigen complexes rather than antibody alone.

Mention has been made above of tumours, since allogeneic transplants of solid tumours evoke a response which closely parallels skin graft rejection. Equally, there is evidence that an individual who spontaneously develops a tumour may mount an immune response against it, despite the fact that the transformed cells are of 'self' origin.

Human cancer patients, for example, sometimes show evidence of cytotoxic antibodies in their circulation, and while these may not greatly influence the growth of a solid tumour, they can be of considerable importance in controlling dispersal and further growth of individual tumour cells (metastasis).

The implication of these observations is that many tumours carry tumour-specific antigens by which they may be recognized as foreign. The nature of these antigens varies according to the origin of the tumour; they may be products of an infecting viral genome, or products of the host genome whose activity is modified during tumour induction (oncogenesis). For example a number of well-characterized tumours show cell-surface antigens which otherwise occur only in the foetus. Normally in adult life these embryonic molecules are suppressed but derepression of the genes concerned results in their expression under abnormal circumstances such as oncogenesis. There is obvious interest in tumour-specific antigens since, if the specific immune response against them could be encouraged, tumour growth could be controlled. In a further parallel with graft rejection, macrophages are involved in the destruction of tumour allografts and, of greater significance, have been implicated in the regression of syngeneic tumour transplants. They are thus able to mediate the response to tumour specific antigens, normally under the influence of T-cell lymphokines. However it has also been shown that agents such as bacterial adjuvants are able to activate macrophages directly in such a way as to heighten their anti-tumour activity. (An adjuvant is a substance whose administration at or around the time of immunization leads to a non-specific enhancement of immune reactivity, so that the particular response under consideration is itself increased.) A further mechanism by which tumour growth or metastasis may be controlled involves natural killer (NK) cells, a population whose relationship to other white blood cells is poorly understood. NK cells show spontaneous cytolytic activity against tumour cells which is independent of pre-immunization or the presence of antibody, and they are thus distinct from K cells.

6.2 Major histocompatibility complexes and the evolution of transplantation immunity

A fruitful offshoot of immunological research has been an increase in our understanding of genetic mechanisms. For instance the study of antibody structure and synthesis has given new insights into the relationships of V- and C-region genes, and therefore into the regulation of protein synthesis in general. Perhaps the best explored area in immunogenetics, in man and mouse at least, is the role of that part of the genome which controls the expression of histocompatibility (transplantation) antigens, the MHC. The MHC in the mouse is known as the H–2 system (= histocompatibility–2, since products of this system were contained in the second of four groups of antigens identified by Gorer as a result of immunizing rabbits with cells from inbred strains of mice). It is found on mouse chromosome 17. In man the MHC is located on chromosome 6 and is known as the HLA system (*h*uman *l*eucocyte group *A* antigens). For a detailed discussion of these systems, see FESTENSTEIN and DÉMANT, 1978. Originally defined because of their

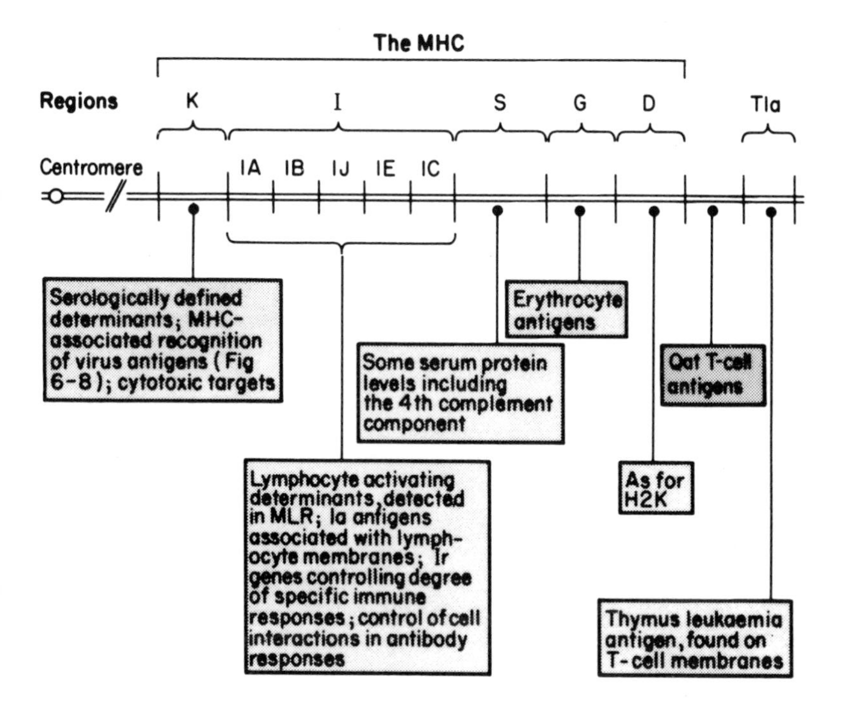

Fig. 6–3 Diagramatic representation of the mouse MHC (H2 system) on chromosome 17, with an indication of the known functional characteristics of the gene products. This information has been obtained due to the ready availability of inbred mouse strains and the identification of certain important recombinants. An MHC with many similar functions is associated with human chromosome 6. It contains genes coding for serologically defined and lymphocyte activating determinants as well as other cell membrane components and is thus of considerable importance in clinical transplantation, and in associated tissue-typing assays. Also associates with the complex are genes controlling the production of C2 and C4. Interest in the human MHC has been greatly stimulated by recent discoveries that a number of diseases are linked to particular HLA genotypes.

importance in determining graft acceptance or rejection, these systems have greatly increased in interest following the discovery that they contain loci which have important immunoregulatory functions (Fig. 6–3).

In the mouse MHC, the K and D regions contain between them three multi-allelic loci. The products of these loci are expressed on the surface of lymphocytes and other cells, and induce good antibody production when mice of one inbred strain are immunized with lymphocytes carrying different K and D alleles. For this reason, K and D products are known as serologically defined determinants, in contradistinction to those products of the MHC which are defined by their ability to activate T-cells in an MLR, and are known as lymphocyte activating determinants (Lad's; see below). Careful analysis of K and D products with suitable antisera indicates that the products of many alleles show immunological cross-reactivity although most of these molecules also have unique determinants. These determinants are known respectively as public and private specificities.

A great deal of present interest in the mouse MHC centres on the I region, for this not only codes for the Lad's, but contains immune-response (Ir) genes which control the level of responsiveness to certain antigens, and also genes whose products, the I region-associated (Ia) antigens, have been linked with the T-cell receptor and other related structures (see Chapter 5). It seems very likely that there will prove to be an overlap between these three classes of molecule, and the product of a single gene may serve in more than one category. One interesting feature of the Lad's is that although the proliferative response in MLRs is due to genetic differences at these loci between target and responder cells, the presence of cytotoxic lymphocytes is not detected unless there are also differences at H–2K or H–2D. The implication of this for allograft rejection is that helper T-cells are required to generate an anti-K or anti-D cytotoxic response, and that these helper cells are stimulated only by I-region products.

The major evolutionary difficulty with graft rejection mechanisms is finding a real explanation for why allografts should be rejected at all, especially since exposure to alloantigens is an unnatural situation for all species except perhaps for colonial organisms such as sponges and some coelenterates. At a superficial level graft rejection is obviously due to the elaborate polymorphism which is associated, in the mouse, with K, I and D regions, and depends on the various gene products being strongly antigenic in genetically different individuals and strains. The distinction between serologically defined determinants and Lad's, particularly in relation to helper T-lymphocyte stimulation, underlines the fact that this is a complex situation, and a good biological reason for existing polymorphisms needs to be provided.

Cell-mediated immunity apparently has a longer evolutionary history than humoral immunity, and it is easier to demonstrate graft rejection in the Agnatha than it is to provoke antibody synthesis. One explanation given for the origin of cell-mediated immunity which received considerable support at one time was that it evolved as a surveillance mechanism, affording protection against the higher incidence of tumours that, it was said, might be associated with the longer lifespan of many vertebrates. A major stumbling block to the general acceptance of this theory proved to be the observation that animals depleted of T-lymphocytes (congenitally or experimentally) failed to develop the rich crop of tumours which was predicted in the absence of the surveillance mechanism. Nonetheless, certain tumours of viral origin do show an increased frequency in such animals and an interesting link between tumour specific antigens and the MHC has been described by Zinkernagel and Doherty. It was shown that viral antigens in the tumour plasma membrane can have a functional relationship with products of H–2D or H–2K, so that the T-cell response to the infected cell required recognition of both the viral and the host component (Fig. 6–4). It is not yet clear whether T-cells possess two separate receptors, one for each component of this dual recognition system, or whether viral antigens can become so closely associated with the MHC product that a single receptor can embrace them both at the same time.

In the light of these relationships, it is possible that polymorphisms at the D and K loci offer selective advantage as a mechanism which limits the possibility of viruses adapting in such a way as to confound the immune response against infected cells. Equally, polymorphisms at other loci, particularly in the I region, could contribute to the flexibility of immune responses, although this would depend on Lad's also having specific function in, say, T-cell recognition mechanisms or T–B interaction. In this respect it is perhaps important to show whether, in allograft rejection, T-cells respond to MHC products because of their inherent involvement in recognition mechanisms or merely because they are different.

6.3 Immunological tolerance

Under certain conditions, exposure to an antigen may lead not to the production of antibodies or to the development of cell-mediated immunity, but to a specific loss of the ability to respond to that particular antigen. This was first recognized as a result of Owen's (1945) studies on non-identical twin cattle. Some such animals are synchorial during foetal life: that is to say, they share the same blood circulation and can exchange circulating cells. These twins then grow up as so-called chimaeras (in Greek mythology, the chimaera was a monster composed

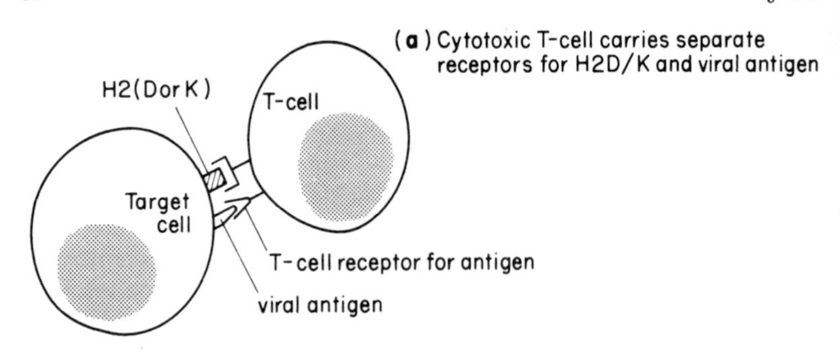

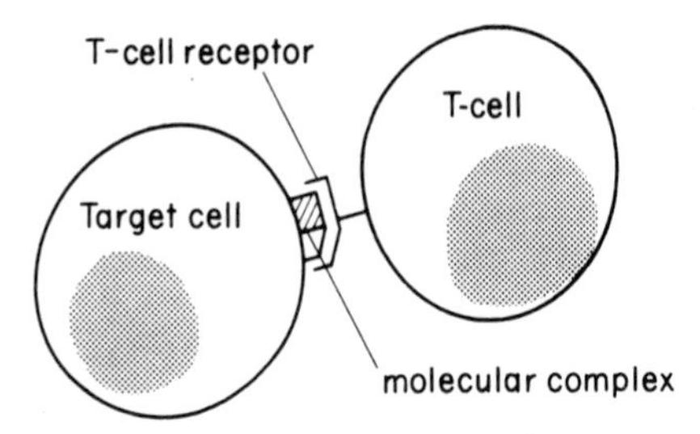

Fig. 6–4 H2 restriction of cytotoxic T-cell response. T-cells can only kill virus-infected target cells if they carry the same H2D or H2K specificity as that carried by the responding cells. This implies that T-lymphocytes carry receptors for all or part of their own H2D/K membrane molecules.

of elements of lion, goat and serpent): more prosaically, they contain cells of two genotypes, their own, and some mobile cells which are derived from the other twin. In adult life, however, no antibodies are formed against the foreign cells, and if skin grafts are exchanged between the twins, they are accepted.

Clearly, such a lack of response would not normally be expected if cells were injected or skin grafted to a genetically foreign individual; the behaviour of the immune system in the cattle twins has evidently been changed as a result of the exposure to foreign cells during foetal life. The change is specific, since a normal immune response is accorded to allografts from a third party. Owen's observations led Burnet to propose that animals would fail to respond to any antigens encountered during prenatal or perhaps early postnatal life: rather, they would 'tolerate' them as if they were part of 'self'.

This important hypothesis soon received support from experiments in which newborn mice were injected with allogeneic cells and subsequently grew up specifically tolerant of donor-strain grafts (Fig. 6–5). Later it turned out that tolerance could be induced to many antigens even in adult life, although whether tolerance, rather than immunity, resulted depended critically upon the dose of antigen and the physical form in which it was administered. With soluble protein antigens, for example, aggregated preparations tended to induce immunity, while material from which all aggregates had been removed by ultracentrifugation or gel filtration induced tolerance. With some weakly immunogenic antigens, such as bovine serum albumin in mice, it was possible to induce tolerance by injecting doses (1–10 μg) too small to evoke immunity. These observations led to the idea that a degree of tolerance induction might be of common occurrence, even with immunogenic doses of antigen, the tolerance being masked by the concomitant induction of immunity. The importance of the physical form of an antigen was explained on the basis that, in order to induce immunity, an antigen required some initial handling by macrophages and that deaggregated proteins were not easily taken up by phagocytic cells.

It is now appreciated that tolerance may be expressed in both T- and B-lymphocyte populations, although that induced by small antigen doses probably affects T-lymphocytes only. Induction of tolerance in B-lymphocytes requires far higher (supra-immunogenic) doses of antigen,

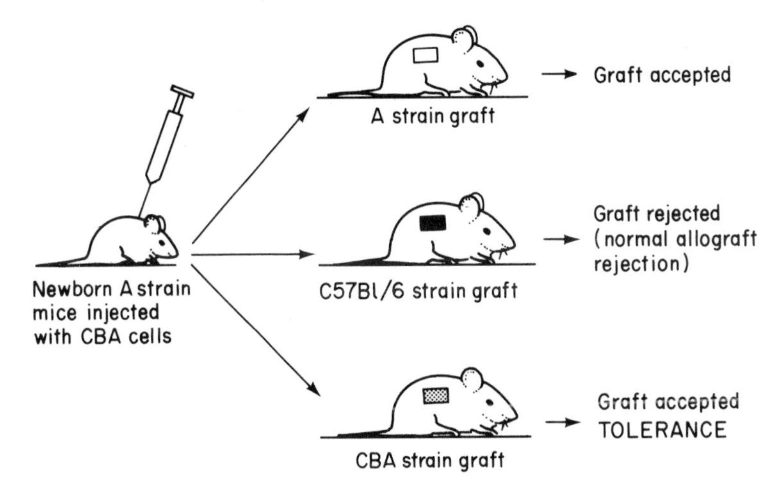

Fig. 6–5 Tolerance induction: CBA skin grafts on adult A strain mice are normally rapidly rejected, but previous injection of CBA strain lymphoid cells into newborn A strain mice renders them tolerant. CBA grafts applied two months later are then accepted.

and under these conditions T-lymphocytes are also rendered tolerant. This was demonstrated by the elegant experiments of Weigle in which combinations of tolerant or normal B- or T-lymphocytes were injected into irradiated recipient mice and challenged with antigen. These experiments also demonstrated, at the level of the whole animal, that recovery from tolerance eventually occurs, and that this is much faster in the B-lymphocyte than in the T-lymphocyte population, reflecting the rates at which new cells are generated in bone marrow and thymus.

Until recently, it was generally assumed that tolerance always reflected the destruction, or at least the irreversible inactivation, of those clones of lymphocyte capable of responding to the antigen in question. It was further assumed that the experimental induction of tolerance mirrored the natural acquisition of tolerance to the potential antigens of 'self'. However, this simple interpretation has been clouded by the discovery of suppressor T-lymphocytes which raised the possibility that reactive clones were not eliminated during tolerance, merely held in check. It has been shown, for instance, that if T-lymphocytes are removed from a functionally tolerant mouse and transferred into irradiated recipients along with normal spleen cells, then the latter population is inhibited from giving a response to the antigen used to generate tolerance in the separate T-lymphocyte population. This sort of effect has been called 'infectious tolerance', and obviously the tolerant T-cells are not all eliminated but alive and well and engaging in suppressor activity. It is apparent, then, that some examples of B-lymphocyte tolerance are due to the activity of suppressor cells. On the other hand, since it usually takes a large dose of antigen to induce suppressors, the kind of tolerance found among T-lymphocytes after low antigen doses is still best attributed to clonal elimination.

With regard to self tolerance, there is growing evidence that an animal's B-lymphocytes may normally be capable of reacting against 'self' and that, if appropriate T-cell help is provided, they may mature to plasmocytes and form autoantibodies. The presumption remains that self-reactive T-cells are normally absent or inactivated. There have been reports of specific anti-graft alloantibodies in animals rendered tolerant to alloantigens at birth, while grafts of skin remain unscathed. This, again, suggests that the T-lymphocytes which could initiate graft rejection have been largely removed by the procedure of tolerance induction, but that B-cells of the same specificity remain.

6.4 Allergic reactions

Hypersensitivity reactions, or allergies, result when an immunological response to an antigen causes the release or activation of pharmacologically active substances which in turn produce unusual and often distressing tissue damage. Symptoms may be localized if exposure to the sensitizing antigen is confined to a small area of the body. On the other hand, if the antigen is more pervasive, as happens with hay fever or some drug allergies for instance, the symptoms can be widespread and, in some sensitive mammalian species, may result in death. Although the benefits usually outweigh the disadvantages, it remains something of a mystery as to why evolution should have produced an immune system with potentially harmful side effects.

It used to be fashionable to divide hypersensitivity reactions on the basis of the speed with which they develop after antigenic challenge. It is now accepted as being more precise and convenient to classify them into four groups according to the type of immunological or pharmacological reaction involved (some additional groups are also recognized). Three of these groups involve the participation of antibody (normally IgE or IgG) while the fourth is essentially a cell-mediated response involving T-lymphocytes alone. However, a degree of overlap between the four categories is often seen. It is a criterion of all four groups that the responding animal has previously been immunized, and thus sensitized, to the offending antigen, and that the physiological symptoms result from a secondary response after re-exposure to the same antigen. Hypersensitivity reactions are distinguished as follows:

Type I Certain antibodies, notably IgE in man and rodents, have the ability to bind via their Fc portions to mast cells in the tissues and mucus membranes. They are collectively known as reaginic antibodies, and, once located in the tissue, they provide a ready trap for antigen following any subsequent challenge. Binding to antigen causes conformational changes in the antibody molecules which lead in turn to rupture of the mast cell membranes and release of vasoactive substances such as histamine and serotonin. Oedema due to increased capillary permeability results, as does contraction of smooth muscle: hence the streaming eyes and nose of hay fever and the respiratory difficulties which are characteristic of asthma or some systemic Type I responses (Fig. 6–6). Systemic reactions can produce very severe symptoms due to the speed at which this category of response can develop and the very small amounts of antigen needed to provoke them.

The evolutionary basis for the manufacture of antibodies with such undesirable properties has been a matter of some debate. However, it has been suggested that smooth muscle spasms are an excellent way of ridding the alimentary tract of unwanted helminths or other parasites, and certainly the vomiting, colonic spasms and diarrhoea which accompany intestinal Type I reactions lend weight to this hypothesis.

Type II Also known as cytotoxic hypersensitivity, this reaction results from the binding of antibody to antigens localized on cell surfaces. Death of the cells usually follows due to the opsonic activity of

(a) IgE manufactured by plasma cells after first exposure to allergen (antigen)
IgE binds via Fc piece to membranes of mast cells in the tissues

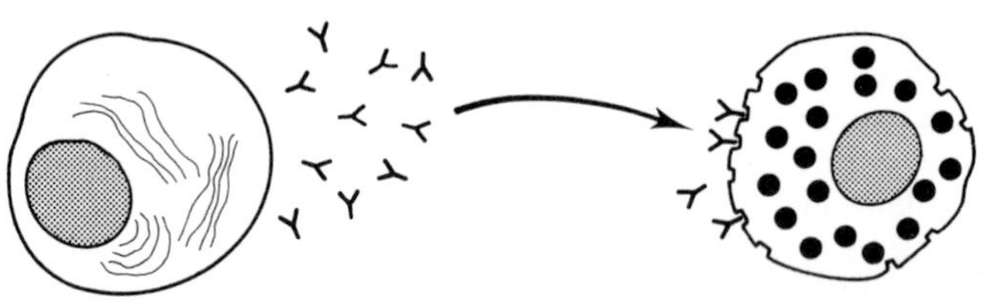

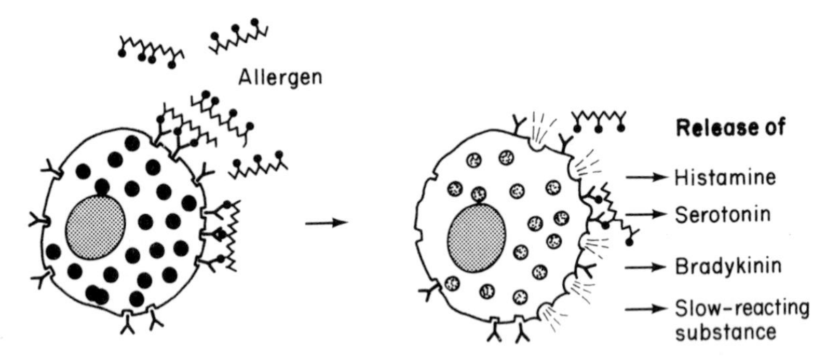

Fig. 6–6 Cellular basis of Type I hypersensitivity reaction, also known as anaphylaxis. Entry of allergens via the respiratory or alimentary tracts can cause severe local symptoms, while if an allergen is introduced systemically, body-wide symptoms can follow. Histamine and serotonin both cause the rapid contraction of certain (but not all) smooth muscles and increase capillary permeability, thus increasing the flow of fluid into the tissues. In addition histamine acts as a vasodilator. Slow-reacting substance (SRS-A) and bradykinin both induce powerful *prolonged* contractions of smooth muscle while bradykinin also increases capillary permeability and has a strong vasodilator activity.

the bound antibodies or as a result of the lytic activity of K-cells or complement, both of which are activated by the antibody component. In humans, Rhesus haemolytic anaemia is an example of this type of reaction. It occurs late in pregnancy in Rh^- mothers bearing an Rh^+

foetus and results from exposure of the mother to foetal erythrocytes which leak across the placenta. Repeated pregnancies can build up high antibody titres, and since maternal IgG can cross the placenta into the foetal circulation, foetal red cells are lysed in the presence of complement. A further example is seen in certain autoimmune diseases, following the manufacture of antibodies against 'self' cells, and it may also occur when drugs bind to cell membranes within the tissues, changing in the process from an innocuous hapten to a fully-fledged and potentially dangerous antigen.

Type III Reactions of this type occur when complexes of antigen and complement-fixing antibody form in the blood or tissues and are not immediately cleared by phagocytic cells. If deposition of these complexes follows, then the activation of complement, and particularly the production of C3a and C5a, results in tissue damage due to histamine release and the degranulation of granulocytes (polymorphonuclear leukocytes) which are chemotactically attracted to the site.

If antigenic challenge is confined to a local site in animals with high antibody titres (Arthus reaction), the symptoms may be similarly localized. On the other hand, if large doses of antigen are introduced systemically, such as happens, say, during passive immunization against tetanus with horse gamma-globulin, then deposition of complexes may occur in the joints, kidneys and other tissues, and widespread damage result. This latter reaction, known as serum sickness, has led to the abandonment of this sort of therapy except as an extreme measure.

Type IV This reaction is often known as delayed-type hypersensitivity, since evidence of the response is not usually manifest for 24–48 hours. The allergic reaction is due to contact between antigen and primed T-lymphocytes, and results from the secretion by the latter of soluble lymphokines which cause local oedema, attract other lymphocytes and macrophages to the site, and increase phagocytic activity. The tissue damage which results, together with the local influx of cells, gives a characteristic induration and erythema if the response takes place in the skin, as for example in forms of contact dermatitis or following the Mantoux (BCG) test for tuberculin sensitivity. In fact, the response to a number of bacterial, viral and fungal infections are characterized by Type IV reactions, particularly where intracellular parasites are involved, and some examples of contact dermatitis also fall into this category.

6.5 Maternal-foetal relationships

During the course of vertebrate evolution, the system of acquired immunity has adapted in the face of a variety of challenges, of which one of the most interesting is presented by the placental mammals. There are obvious advantages in viviparity for warm-blooded, terrestrial animals, but the evolution of the placenta has inevitably resulted in the presentation to the pregnant female of paternal (allogeneic) antigens on the foetus. We should expect the mammalian foetus to be rejected; indeed the potential hazards of pregnancy are well illustrated by the phenomenon of Rhesus haemolytic disease in man, mentioned in the previous section, where leakage into Rh^- females of Rh^+ foetal erythrocytes leads to antibody formation and resultant anaemia or death in the foetus.

The immunological background to the survival of the mammalian foetus in normal circumstances is again something of a mystery. Undoubtedly in some animals, for instance the pig, the epithelio-chorial placenta acts as an effective barrier between mother and foetus. Here the embryonic trophoblast and chorion are apposed to the epithelium of the uterine wall. There is no direct contact between foetal tissues and the maternal circulation, and only nutrients are able to pass across. In such species, the young rely for their own early protection on antibodies in the mother's milk rather than the passage of maternal antibodies across the placenta. On the other hand, in many other species, invasion of the uterine wall by embryonic tissues occurs, and in the haemo-chorial placenta of rodents and primates, the trophoblast is bathed by the maternal blood. In this situation there is clear evidence of antigenic material, including viable foetal cells, entering the mother's circulation, and antibodies against foetal antigens are commonly found in pregnant females.

It follows from the above that some modulation of the effector arm of the immune system must occur during pregnancy in many mammalian species, and a number of mechanisms have been proposed. It has been suggested, for instance, that the embryonic tissue in closest contact with the mother, the trophoblast, has its cell surface antigens partially concealed below a layer of mucopolysaccharide rich in sialic acid, and also that these antigens are sparsely distributed. Thus efficient contact of cytotoxic lymphocytes with the trophoblast surface might be prevented. It should be noted, however, that, following endometrial cup formation in the Equidae, where isolated groups of large trophoblast cells develop in the uterine wall, invasion of the embryonic tissue by maternal lymphocytes takes place. Endometrial cup degeneration in these situations is associated with increased lymphocyte invasion. If, on the other hand, the trophoblast proper is protected from contact with maternal T-cells, then anti-foetal antibodies might act as blocking factors, and work in conjunction with the mucopolysaccharide layer to conceal the trophoblast antigens. Antibodies acting in this way would be analogous to the enhancing antibodies which prolong the survival of tumours and allogeneic tissue grafts. Protection of the foetus itself from these antibodies might be due to a mechanism such as that recently proposed whereby cells with Fc receptors, situated in the body of the placenta, absorb out antibodies or antibody–antigen complexes, and prevent complement-dependent tissue damage in the embryo.

There is also evidence that the immune mechanisms of pregnant mammals are suppressed, and that such responses as do occur are weak when compared with those to allogeneic antigens in non-pregnant females. In a variety of assays, including mixed lymphocyte reactions, lymphocyte response to mitogens, allograft rejection and contact sensitivity, evidence for the suppression of cell-mediated responses in particular has accumulated, although the precise nature of the suppression is not certain. Humoral factors associated with pregnancy, especially HCG and alpha-foetoprotein, have been shown to have immunosuppressive properties, and it may also be the case that suppressor T-lymphocytes are more active during pregnancy, particularly in lymphoid organs draining the uterus.

It is clear that the mammalian foetus is antigenically mature in that it expresses paternal alloantigens from a very early stage in development, and also, in many species, that pregnant females are exposed to foetal antigens or cells. The eventual survival of the foetus is probably due to a variety of protective mechanisms working in combination, some of which will be superfluous in situations like the pig, where the placenta itself is a simple and effective barrier. In other mammals, where the placenta has evolved and become more efficient, particularly in the area of protective immunity by allowing passage of maternal antibodies, there is also increased risk of immunological rejection of the foetus. In these conditions, the different factors outlined above combine to ensure its survival.

7 The Future

It is perhaps justifiable to wonder where all the present activity in immunology is leading us. Some trends do seem to be discernible. For convenience we can consider them under three categories, although, as will shortly be apparent, items in the different categories may be related to each other.

7.1 Practical benefits

7.1.1 Parasitic diseases

Immunological research during the early decades of this century have had a profound effect on human (and animal) health, leading to the virtual elimination of some infectious diseases such as smallpox and the possibility of providing resistance to many others. However, there are groups of infectious diseases on which immunology has so far made only a negligible impact. These are the diseases caused by parasitic protozoa and helminths. They are of immense social and economic importance, particularly in less developed parts of the world, and non-immunological attempts to combat them have so far largely failed. On the face of it, the immune system should be well equipped to deal with such invaders, and a degree of immunity may eventually result from natural infections. But there are problems: vaccines have generally not proved to be useful, and organisms such as trypanosomes (which cause sleeping sickness and allied diseases in man and animals) appear adept at changing their surface antigens and hence keeping one jump ahead of the immune response. Other parasites contrive to produce a general immunosuppression in their hosts. It is only very recently that the immunology of parasitic diseases has begun to attract anything like its fair share of attention, and work in this field can be expected to intensify.

7.1.2 Cancer

Few people doubt that close links exist between the immune system and processes of neoplasia (the induction, development and control of cancer). Indeed, the hypothesis of immunological surveillance which, although less popular now, has been influential over several years, holds that the main *raison d'être* of the immune system is to detect and eliminate cells carrying unusual antigens on their surface. It is certain that many experimentally-induced tumours in animals carry such tumour specific antigens and can evoke an immune response by the host. However, great caution has to be used in extrapolating from these results, particularly since similar antigens have rarely been identified on tumours that arise 'spontaneously' in man. Another reason is that the intervention of the immune system can lead to enhancement or facilitation of the growth of a tumour rather than to its elimination as happens, for example, when antibodies against a tumour block the response of cytotoxic T-cells. A resolute feeling still persists that manipulation of the immune system will eventually turn out to be the key to the successful treatment of many human tumours, and immunotherapy is already practiced in some cases, but hopes that a major 'breakthrough' may be imminent seem if anything to have receded during the last few years.

7.1.3 Development studies

Finally mention should be made of an application of immunology which, although not providing any immediate practical benefits to mankind, is of great scientific interest and may well provide practical benefits in the future: this is in the study of cell and tissue differentiation. It is becoming clear, particularly from extensive studies of lymphocytes (section 3.1), that cells which differ functionally, or are at different stages along a differentiation pathway, have distinct and specific chemical structures in their cell membranes. These may be recognized as antigenic by animals of another species (or even, on occasion, of the same species) and antibodies may be prepared against them. Such antibodies can be used to tag cells carrying the specific antigens either *in vivo* or *in vitro* or, in conjunction with complement, to kill them. There is no reason to doubt that other cells besides lymphocytes will repay study by such methods. So far, a major problem has been that animals tend to produce a variety of antibodies when they are immunized, in addition to those directed against the particular determinant in which one is interested. These other antibodies may react with a wide range of cell types and have to be removed by absorption before a specific antiserum can be obtained – a process which is often laborious and inefficient. However, this approach to developmental biology will be revolutionized by the recently developed techniques for producing large amounts of monospecific antibody (see below). These techniques are already producing antibodies of far greater potency and discriminating power than have previously been available.

7.2 Ideas

In the relatively short history of immunology, quite a small number of ideas can be identified as having had a pre-eminent influence on the course of research. Burnet's clonal selection theory of 1957 was one such. More recently, the theory of immune surveillance, referred to above, has also had a pervasive, although less significant, influence.

A set of ideas which seems likely to have a dominating influence on immunology during the next few years is that encompassed under the heading of 'network' theories, as introduced particularly by Jerne. From the outset, some aspects of network theory were perhaps more firmly founded on experimental observations than, at their inception, were either clonal selection or immune surveillance, more indeed than immune surveillance has ever been. Jerne's proposal draws together two well-established facts: first, that lymphocytes carry receptors for antigen on their surface; second, the existence of idiotypes which, it will be remembered, are antigenic specificities associated with the variable region of an Ig molecule. It follows that a virgin population of lymphocytes will carry a cumulatively large array of potentially antigenic idiotypes. When a particular clone of lymphocytes is stimulated by exposure to antigen, the amount of that clone's idiotype will increase greatly and may in principle evoke an immune response. It can readily be seen that the cells responding to the idiotype will themselves carry an idiotype of their own which in turn might evoke an immune response. The process could in principle be never-ending, but in practice would doubtless be limited by the decreasing size of each sequential stimulus and hence of the response evoked, until the stimulus was no longer immunogenic. A further fact, with which the reader will already be familiar, must be drawn into the argument at this stage: that is the phenomenon of cross-reaction. Like any other antibodies, anti-idiotypic antibodies would be expected to react not only with the idiotype that evoked them, but with other idiotypic determinants of related shape and possibly also with some exogenous antigens. The consequences of introducing an antigen into such a system can be seen to be far-reaching. As Raff has aptly put it, antigen may induce 'a reverberating perturbation of the network', rather than the simple response of individual antigen-sensitive lymphocytes which is commonly envisaged. The components of this network are shown in a simple form in Fig. 7–1. If, as has been suggested, anti-idiotypic responses exercise a suppressive effect on idiotype-bearing clones, the system can provide an elegant mechanism for homeostatic regulation of antibody responses via negative feed-back. Figure 7–1 is depicted in terms of B-lymphocytes and antibodies only; further dimensions of complexity are added by the participation of T-lymphocytes in all their diversity and perhaps also, by virtue of their cytophilic antibody, macrophages.

Since the response to a normal antigenic stimulus involves many clones of cells, one might think that it would be almost impossible to provide any experimental verification of these ideas. However, certain

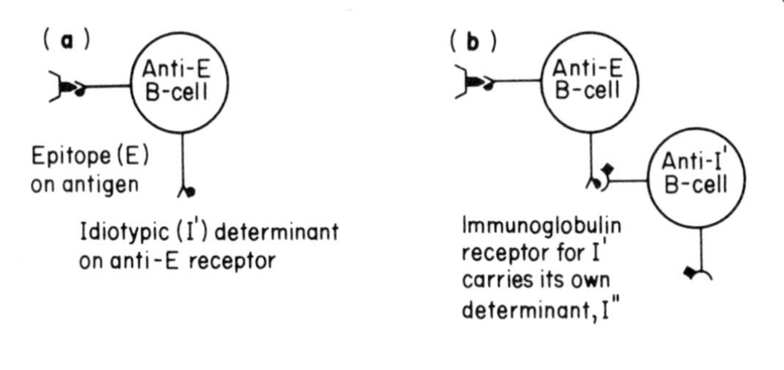

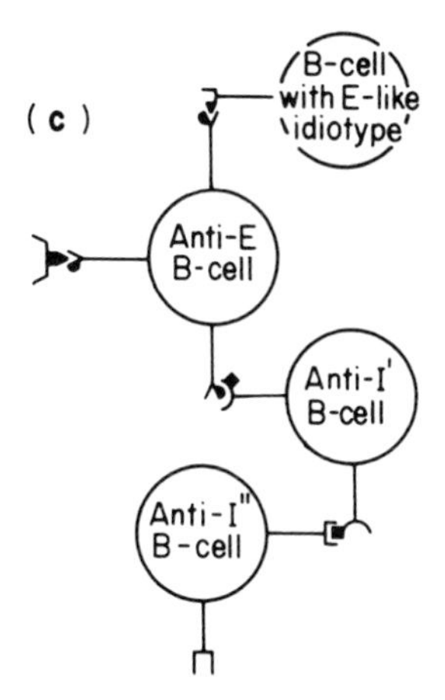

Fig. 7–1 Illustration of some of the interactions which are predicted by Jerne's network theory. It is suggested that interactions such as these impose self-regulatory constraints on the immune system.

antigens, such as phosphorylcholene in mice, evoke a homogeneous response consisting of antibodies largely of a single idiotype. With this antigen, it has proved possible to demonstrate the appearance of an anti-idiotypic response and its influence on the response to the original antigen.

As the whole picture becomes clearer, it will probably turn out that helper and suppressor T-cells recognize B-cells and each other by means of a complex network of idiotype/anti-idiotype reactions, and that this network is the basis for the initiation and regulation of any immune response. It seems safe to predict that network theories will continue to be a strong influence in immunology over the next few years.

7.3 Techniques

As mentioned above, antibodies are of enormous potential value in analysing and classifying the surfaces of cells, and in separating cells on the basis of their membrane antigenicity. Antibodies have already been much used in this way for the study of the component parts of the immune system itself. What is ideally wanted for such work is a collection of antibodies, each of a single specificity. Rapidly growing malignant clones of antibody-forming cells would be perfect for producing these. Such malignant tumours do indeed exist in some species, including mouse, rat and man; they are known as myelomas or plasmacytomas, and produce large quantities of homogeneous immunoglobulin. Unfortunately, the antibody specificity of this immunoglobulin is rarely identifiable, and attempts to induce myelomas of known specificity in hyper-immunized animals have been unsuccessful. It has recently proved possible, however, to fuse myeloma cells with normal cells producing specific antibody. A proportion of the hybrid daughter cells carry all the desirable characteristics of both parents: that is, they grow rapidly and continuously *in vitro* or *in vivo*, producing large quantities of immunoglobulin, and this immunoglobulin is of the same specificity as that produced by the normal (non-tumorous) parent cell. By means of a series of reasonably simple technical manipulations *in vitro*, individual rapidly proliferating clones of cells can be isolated, each of which produces 'monoclonal' antibody of a single specificity. Such clones can be maintained for considerable periods, or even indefinitely, and large amounts of their antibody product can be harvested. It must be re-emphasized that, however complex the antigen used for initial immunization of the animal from which the normal parent of the hybrid came, the antibody made by each clone will react with only one single determinant and with uniform affinity. In this way, large collections of monospecific antibodies can be built up against any antigens required. For the first time, it is possible to exploit to the full the exquisite discriminatory power of the immune system to analyse complex mixtures of antigens such as are present on the cell surface. This process is only just beginning, but is gathering pace rapidly. Already, most sizeable laboratories of experimental immunology are engaged in the production and maintenance of 'hybridomas' for one purpose or another, and monoclonal antibodies to some antigens, including Thy-1 and mouse Ig delta chains, are being used routinely. Nor is the usefulness of cell-fusion techniques in immunology confined to the production of monospecific antibodies. Recent experiments indicate that it is also possible to fuse T-lymphocytes of a given specificity and function with appropriate T-type tumour cells (lymphomas).

Another recent technical innovation which will be increasingly used by cellular immunologists during the coming years is the fluorescence-activated cell sorter. This instrument analyses and separates cells on the basis of their fluorescence. From the immunologist's point of view, the most useful way to induce fluorescence is to label the cells with antibody to one or more of the membrane constituents and to tag these antibodies with a fluorochrome such as fluorescein or rhodamine. Thus, cells which carry a particular antigenic determinant can be separated from those that do not, and it is even possible to separate cells carrying high and low concentrations of the determinant. The essential features of the cell sorter are shown in Fig. 7–2. The cells are made to pass one by one

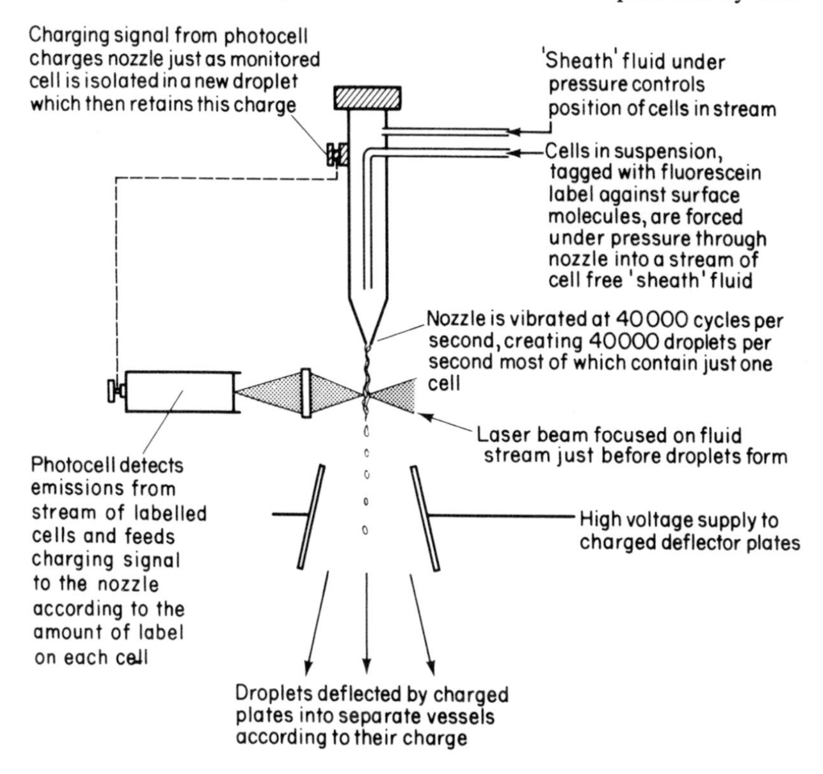

Fig. 7–2 The fluorescence-activated cell sorter is already making a considerable impact on immunological research owing to its ability to produce suspensions which are greatly enriched for one particular cell type, provided that the cell has a distinct cell surface marker which can be labelled with a fluorescent antibody. Actual separation depends on the charge conferred on each individual droplet, but the key operation is ensuring that only the correct droplets are charged (apparatus drawn from HERZENBERG L. A. *et al*, 1976).

through a laser beam, and one or more fluorescence detectors register the light emitted from each cell. The optical signals are translated into electrical pulses which are processed and stored for display and analysis. When the cells are to be sorted, as opposed to merely analysed, the stream of cells is subjected to ultrasonic vibration which causes it to break up into minute droplets (40 000 per second) at a fixed distance below the detection point. Thus each cell becomes enclosed, usually by itself, in a droplet. While the cell is passing from the detection point to the tip of the stream, its fluorescence output is processed and compared with preset parameters determining which of two subpopulations it should be assigned to. Application of an electrical charge to the stream at the moment the cell reaches the tip of the stream charges the appropriate droplet and charged deflecting plates subsequently direct it into one or other of two receptacles. Uncharged droplets continue directly downwards into a third receptacle. Despite its considerable expense, this instrument is appearing in an increasing number of laboratories. Obviously, the results obtained can only be as good as the antibodies used to tag the cells in the first place. Here, monospecific hybrid-derived antibodies really come into their own, and their existence will enormously increase the scope and usefulness of the cell sorter. The instrument described does in fact also sort on the basis of forward angle light scatter (broadly a measurement of particle or cell size), so that the operator can select any combination of size and fluorescence intensity that he wishes.

The reader who has persevered this far will have little difficulty in imagining the range of experiments which will be made possible by combining these sorts of technique.

Further Reading

Books

FESTENSTEIN, H. and DÉMANT, P. (1978). *HLA and H-2: Basic Immunogenetics, Biology and Clinical Relevance*. Current Topics in Immunology, volume **9**; Edward Arnold, London.

FUDENBERG, H. H., PINK, J. R. L., WANG, A-C. and DOUGLAS, S. D. (1978). *Basic Immunogenetics*, 2nd edition. Oxford University Press, New York.

GOLUB, E. S. (1977). *The Cellular Basis of the Immune Response*. Sinauer Associates, Inc., Sunderland, Mass.

HESLOP-HARRISON, J. (1978). *Cellular Recognition Systems*. Studies in Biology no. 100. Edward Arnold, London.

LOOR, F. and ROELANTS, G. E. (eds) (1977). *B and T cells in Immune Recognition*. John Wiley and Sons, London.

MANNING, M. J. and TURNER, R. J. (1976). *Comparative Immunobiology*. Blackie, Glasgow and London.

MARCHALONIS, J. J. (1977). *Immunity in Evolution*. Edward Arnold, London.

ROITT, I. (1977). *Essential Immunology*, 3rd edition. Blackwell, Oxford.

STEWARD, M. W. (1974). *Immunochemistry*. Chapman and Hall, London.

WEIR, D. M. (1977). *Immunology: An Outline for Students of Medicine and Biology*, 4th edition. Churchill Livingstone, Edinburgh.

Reviews and Other Articles

BACH, F. H., BACH, M. L. and SONDEL, P. M. (1976). Differential function of major histocompatibility complex antigens in T-lymphocyte activation. *Nature*, **259**, 273–81.

BEER, A. E. and BILLINGHAM, R. E. (1974). The embryo as a transplant. *Scientific American*, **230** (April), 36–46.

BLOOM, B. R. (1979). Games parasites play: how parasites evade immune surveillance. *Nature*, **279**, 21–6.

CAPRA, J. D. and EDMUNDSON, A. B. (1977). The antibody combining site. *Scientific American*, **236** (January), 50–9.

CUNNINGHAM, B. A. (1977). The structure and function of histocompatibility antigens. *Scientific American*, **237** (October), 96–107.

EDELMAN, G. M. (1970). The structure and function of antibodies. *Scientific American*, **223** (August), 34–42.

FELDMANN, M. and NOSSAL, G. J .V. (1972). Tolerance, enhancement and the regulation of interaction between T cells, B cells and macrophages. *Transplantation Reviews*, **13**, 3–34.

FORD, W. L. (1975). Lymphocyte migration and immune responses. *Progress in Allergy*, **19**, 1–59.

GIVOL, D. (1976). A structural basis for molecular recognition. The antibody case.

In *Receptors and recognition*, Series A, Vol. 2, P. Cuatrecasas and M. F. Greaves (eds). Chapman and Hall, London, pp. 1–42.

HERZENBERG, L. A., SWEET, R. G. and HERZENBERG, L. A. (1976). Fluorescence-activated cell sorting. *Scientific American*, **234** (March), 108–17.

JERNE, N. K. (1973). The immune system. *Scientific American*, **229** (July), 52–60.

KLEIN, J. (1979). The major histocompatibility complex of the mouse. *Science*, **203**, 516–21.

MAYER, M. M. (1973). The complement system. *Scientific American*, **229** (November), 54–66.

MILLER, J. F. A. P. (1972). Lymphocyte interactions in antibody responses. *International Review of Cytology*, **33**, 77–130.

MUNRO, A. (1978). Interactions between cells of a syngeneic immune system involving products of the major histocompatibility complex. *Proceedings of the Royal Society of London*, Series B, **202**, 177–89.

MUNRO, A. and BRIGHT, S. (1976). Products of the major histocompatibility complex and their relationship to the immune response. *Nature*, **264**, 145–52.

OLD, L. J. (1977). Cancer immunology. *Scientific American*, **236** (May), 62–79.

PAUL, W. E. and BENACERRAF, B. (1977). Functional specificity of thymus-dependent lymphocytes. *Science*, **195**, 1293–300.

PORTER, R. R. (1967). The structure of antibodies. *Scientific American*, **217** (October), 81–90.

RAFF, M. (1977). Immunological networks. *Nature*, **265**, 205–7.